The Sirtfood Diet Cookbook

115 Delicious Recipes to Lose Weight, Reduce Waistlines, Get Toned and Achieve Breathtaking Results!

PATRICIA GARNER

PUBLISHED BY: Green Book Publishing LTD

© Copyright 2020 by Patricia Garner - All rights reserved.

The following eBook is reproduced below with the goal of providing information that is as accurate and reliable as possible.

This declaration is deemed fair and valid by both the American Bar Association and the Committee of Publishers Association and is legally binding throughout the United States.

Furthermore, the transmission, duplication or reproduction of any of the following work including specific information will be considered an illegal act irrespective of if it is done electronically or in print. This extends to creating a secondary or tertiary copy of the work or a recorded copy and is only allowed with the express written consent from the Publisher. All additional right reserved.

Additionally, the information in the following pages is intended only for informational purposes and should thus be thought of as universal. As befitting its nature, it is presented without assurance regarding its prolonged validity or interim quality.

Table of Contents

Introduction 6

What is the Sirtfood Diet? 7

Top Sirtfoods 9
Fruit 9
Vegetables 10
Other 10

RECIPES 11

Breakfast and Smoothies 11
Sirtfood Green Juice 11
Lime and Ginger Green Smoothie 14
Turmeric Strawberry Green Smoothie 16
Sirtfood Wonder Smoothie 18
Strawberry Spinach Smoothie 20
Berry Turmeric Smoothie 22
Mango Green Smoothie 24
Apple Avocado Smoothie 26
Kale Pineapple Smoothie 28
Blueberry Banana Avocado Smoothie 30
Carrot Smoothie 32
Matcha Berry Smoothie 34
Date & Walnut Porridge 36
Sirtfood Breakfast Scramble 38
Simple Grape Smoothie 40
Ginger Plum Smoothie 42
Kumquat Mango Smoothie 44
Cranberry Smoothie 46
Blackberry Banana Smoothie 48
Creamy Pineapple Cucumber Smoothie 50
Carrot Celery Orange & Ginger Smoothie 52
Strawberry Orange Juice 54
Tropical Watercress Juice 56
Arugula Apple Smoothie 58
Sirtfood Omelette 60
Sirtfood Chocolate Strawberry Milk 62
Cranberry & Orange Granola 64
Creamy Coconut Porridge 66
Homemade Muesli 68
Fresh Herbs and Cheese Scramble 70
Dark Chocolate Almond Bars 72
Coconut Yogurt Waffles 74
Cinnamon Buckwheat Bowls 76

Light Bites 78

Sirtfood Salmon Salad 78
Broccoli Salad 80
Buckwheat Stir Fry with Kale, Peppers & Artichokes 83
Arugula, Egg, and Charred Asparagus Salad 86
Spring Vegetable and Quinoa Salad with Bacon 88
Golden Chicory in Prosciutto Wraps 90
Vegetable Cabbage Soup 92
Fresh Herb Frittata 94
Grilled Asparagus with Caper Vinaigrette 96
Herby Pork with Apple & Chicory Salad 98
Chia, Quinoa & Avocado Salad 100
Tomato Green Bean Soup 103
Kale Salad with Pecorino and Lemon 105
Tahini-Date Salted Caramels 107
Bacon-Wrapped Dates 109
Avocado Tuna Salad 111
Herb-Roasted Olives and Tomatoes 113
Roasted Red Onions Stuffed with Mascarpone Cheese 115
Mixed Olive Crostini 117
Cannellini Bean Soup 119
Celery Caesar Salad 121
Orange, Almond & Date Salad 123
Walnut and Onion Tartine 125
Olives and Avocado Salad with Tomatoes and Feta Cheese 127
Crispy Artichoke Hearts with Horseradish Sauce 129

Main Meals 131
Buckwheat & Asparagus Risotto 131
Foil Baked Salmon 133
Crispy Chicken with Sweet Chili Rice 135
Macaroni & Cheese with Broccoli 137
Baked Tofu 139
Fish Taco Cabbage Bowl 141
Asian Chicken Thighs 144
Roast Quail with Rosemary, Thyme and Garlic 146
Garlic Butter Roast Turkey 148
Baked Lemon Butter Tilapia 151
Fried Sardines with Olives 153
Salmon Curry 155
Fish Casserole with Mushrooms and French Mustard 157
Chicken Chili 160
Garlic & Rosemary Grilled Lamb Chops 162
Indian Spiced Cauliflower Rice 164
Cheesy Asparagus 166
Garlic Butter Shrimp 168
Ground Beef & Broccoli 170
Garlic Mushrooms 172

Appetizers & Snacks 174
Broccoli Cheddar Bites 174
No Bake Zucchini Roll-Ups 176

Avocado Deviled Eggs 178
Spicy Deviled Eggs 180
Spicy Roasted Nuts 182
Crab Salad Stuffed Avocado 184
Cheddar Olives 186
Crispy Breaded Tofu Nuggets 188
Rosemary Toasted Walnuts 190
Cream Cheese Stuffed Celery 192
Baked Artichoke & Cilantro Pizza Dipping Sauce 194
Herbed Soy Snacks 196

Desserts 197
Cinnamon & Cardamom Bombs 197
Blueberry Cupcakes 199
Chocolate Cake with Chocolate Glaze 202
Coconut Strawberry Mousse 204
Avocado Popsicles 206
Cheesecake with Blueberries 208
Coconut Lime Bars 210
Chocolate Cookies 212
Pistachio Pudding 214
Apple Berry Crumble Pies 216
Mocha Truffle Cheesecake 218
Vanilla Cheesecake Popsicles 220
Balsamic Plum Ice Cream 222
Frozen Strawberry Yogurt 224
Raspberry-Lemon Cream Cake 226

Dressings 228
Spicy Lemon Herb Sauce 228
Shallots & Red Wine Sauce 230
Italian Mayonnaise 232
Thai Peanut Sauce 234
Cream Cheese with Herbs 236
Avocado Caesar Dressing 238
Mild Curry Seasoning 240
Tzatziki 242
Guacamole 244
Salsa Verde 246

21-Day Meal Plan 248
Conclusion 256

Introduction

Hello and welcome to this amazing guide! The goal of the book is to give you the knowledge of what the Sirtfood Diet is and how it works, why it will work for you, and of course, so many delicious recipes to enjoy!

If you bought this book, you probably want to lose weight, burn fat, get toned, or maybe you want to fix your digestive disorders. There could be so many reasons to start the Sirtfood Diet and each of them is valuable. This program will help you achieving all these goals without any doubt.

I have always been so passionate about healthy eating and diets in general. I believe that health starts from food. That's why I have studied (and followed) so many diets over the last 15 years. I can honestly tell you that the Sirtfood Diet is the one that made me achieve the best results ever! I lost over 10 pounds in the last 3 months. I feel so great and grateful that I want to share my knowledge and my experience to encourage you achieving the results you dream!

I remember how anxious I was when I started the Sirtfood Diet. I wanted to get results so bad! I wanted to look great, to feel confident about myself and be healthy! I achieved all these results, and I'm sure you will too! I can promise that if you follow the program and don't give up, you will get breathtaking results!

In this book, we will mainly focus on recipes, but first we will look at the basics of the Sirtfood Diet to understand its principles. We will keep it simple, because simplicity always pays off!

I wrote another book about Sirtfood Diet that goes much deeper in its foundational aspects and scientifically basements. Therefore, I believe the combination of the two books will give you deep knowledge and terrific results! To get the most complete experience and to get the most out of this diet, take advantages of both books.

Are you ready to start? Enjoy this amazing journey!

What is the Sirtfood Diet?

The Sirtfood Diet is a dietary regime with the characteristic of not excluding any food, and promoting the consume of plant-based foods.

These foods contain polyphenols that activate and stimulate the production of specific proteins, **sirtuins**, which are capable to promote weight loss and gain muscle mass (or at least maintaining it) by activating the "skinny gene".

Basically, when you nosh on the rich-in-sirtuin ingredients, you stimulate the proteins encoded by the SIRT1 gene, known as the skinny gene.

Sirtuins are effective metabolism regulators that influence the ability to burn fat, stabilize mood and the mechanism on which longevity depends.

Sirtuins have many functions:

- Protecting cells from dying when they are under stress.
- Regulate metabolic processes related to insulin resistance.
- They have immunity control.
- They play a fundamental role in epigenetics.
- Protecting against cancer.
- Regulate inflammations and aging processes.

Sirtuins are believed to influence the body's ability to burn fat and boost the metabolism, while maintaining muscles.

The Sirtfood Diet is divided into two phases. The first phase lasts 1 week, which is divided in other 2 phases. The second phase lasts 14 days and has less restrictions than the first.

The first Phase: As I said previously, the first phase lasts only 7 days. The first three days of the week involve restricting calories to 1000 kcal, consuming **3** Sirtfood green juices and **1** solid meal rich in sirtuin each day. In this phase, I take the first green juice at breakfast, the second in the mid-morning and the last one in the afternoon. At dinner, I consume the solid meal. These juices include green tea, lemon, rocket, parsley, kale, berries etc.

Solid meals include turkey, chicken, fish, salad etc.

The second phase of this first week lasts four days. Energy intakes are increased to 1500 kcal, and we will consume **2** Sirtfood green juices and **2** solid sirtuin-rich meals each day. The Sirtfood Diet is very restrictive in your daily calories during the first week, but don't worry, you know why you're doing this so keep on following it!

The second Phase: The second phase lasts 14 days and it is known as the **maintenance phase**. Here we will consume **1** Sirtfood green juice and **3** solid meals. There is no specific calorie restriction for this phase.

Focusing on weight loss is not what the diet is all about! Here we learn to think long term, we integrate these foods in our daily routine to maintain our weight and to stay healthy. This is a very important aspect: you need this diet to be part of your life. It's a lifestyle! The Sirtfood Diet is designed to give you the best foods nature has to offer you, and is sustainable because of its inclusion method, not exclusion. This means that the Sirtfood Diet is compatible to our modern-day living and lifestyle. Anyway, after 90 days maintenance you can repeat the two phases for more weight loss.

Top Sirtfoods

- Arugula (Rocket)
- Kale
- Onion
- Buckwheat
- Parsley
- Red Chicory
- Coffee
- Extra Virgin Olive Oil
- Soy
- Tofu products
- Matcha Green Tea
- Dark Chocolate (80-90% cocoa)
- Olives
- Turmeric
- Strawberries
- Capers
- Red Wine
- Chili (Bird's eye variety)
- Walnuts
- Medjool Dates
- Celery

Fruit

- Strawberries
- Blueberries
- Cranberries
- Blackberries
- Raspberries
- Apple
- Grapes (Red)
- Plums
- Kumquats

Vegetables

- Broccoli
- Asparagus
- Artichokes
- White Onions
- Lettuce
- Shallots
- Yellow Chicory
- Green Beans
- Cabbage

Other

- Ginger
- Peppermint
- Quinoa
- Sunflower Seeds
- Chia Seeds
- Broad Beans
- Chestnuts
- Chili Peppers
- Chives
- Oregano
- Pistachios
- Peanuts
- Cannellini Beans
- Dill
- Sage
- Garlic

RECIPES

Breakfast and Smoothies

Sirtfood Green Juice

This is the famous Sirtfood Green Juice! A delicious and energy-boosting Sirtfood green smoothie!

Ingredients: 1 serving
- 1/3 cup arugula (rocket)
- 2 cups kale
- 1 tablespoon lovage leaves
- 1 tablespoon flat leaf parsley
- ½ teaspoon matcha green tea
- ½ lemon, juiced
- ½ apple
- Large stalks green celery, including leaves

Directions:

- Mix the greens (rocket, kale, parsley and lovage leaves) together, then juice them to get 50ml of juice from the green.

- Juice the apple and the celery.

- You can peel the lemon and put it through the juicer, or simply squeeze the lemon by hand into the juice. You should have 250ml of juice in total by this stage.

- When the juice is made and ready to serve, add the matcha green tea. Pour a small amount of juice into a glass, then add the matcha and stir vigorously with a fork or a teaspoon. (Use matcha only in the first two drinks of the day as it contains moderate amount of caffeine)

- Once the matcha is dissolved add the remainder of the juice. Give it a final stir.

- Enjoy!

Nutritional info per serving: Calories 90, Fat 0g, Carbohydrates 20g, Protein 2g

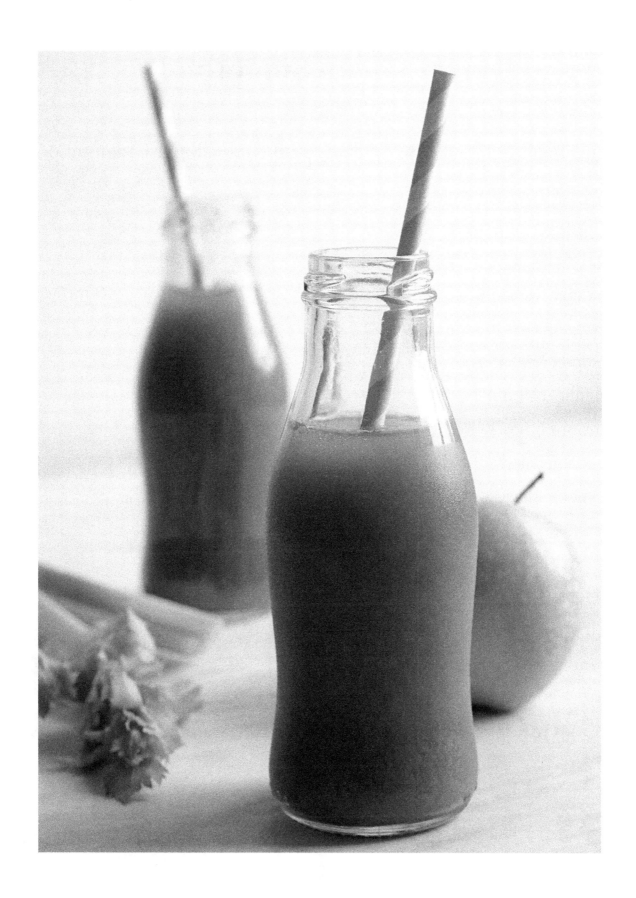

Lime and Ginger Green Smoothie

Taste this healthy, fresh, and amazing Lime and Ginger Green Smoothie!

Ingredients: 1 serving
- ½ cup dairy free milk
- ½ cup water
- ½ teaspoon fresh ginger
- ½ cup mango chunks
- Juice from 1 lime
- 1 tablespoon dried shredded coconut
- 1 tablespoon flaxseeds
- 1 cup spinach

Directions:
- Blend together all the ingredients until smooth.
- Serve and enjoy!

Nutritional info per serving: Calories 178, Fat 1g, Carbohydrates 7g, Protein 4g

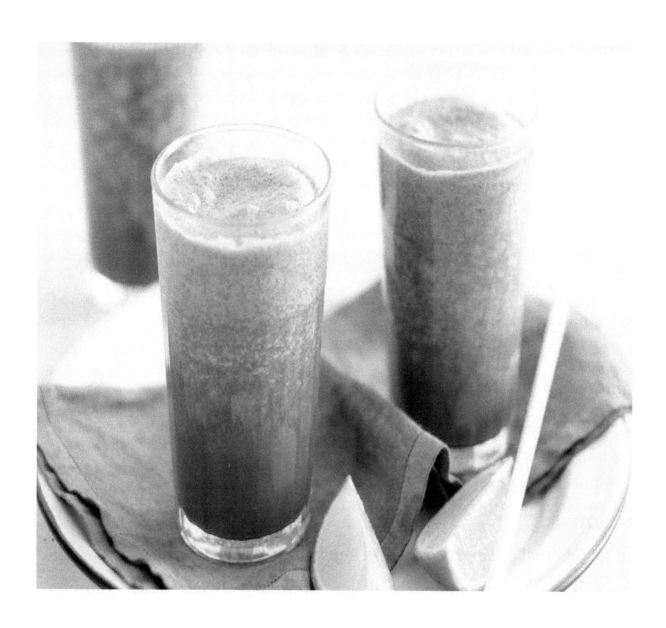

Turmeric Strawberry Green Smoothie

This simple smoothie will help your digestion! Too good not to try it!

Ingredients: 1 serving

- 1 cup kale, stalks removed
- 1 teaspoon turmeric
- 1 cup strawberries
- ½ cup coconut yogurt
- 6 walnut halves
- 1 tablespoon raw cacao powder
- 1-2 mm slice of bird's eye chili
- 1 cup unsweetened almond milk
- 1 pitted Medjool date

Directions:

- Blend together all the ingredients and enjoy immediately!
- Be careful how much almond milk you add so you can choose your favourite consistency.

Nutritional info per serving: Calories 180, Fat 2.2g, Carbohydrates 12g, Protein 4g

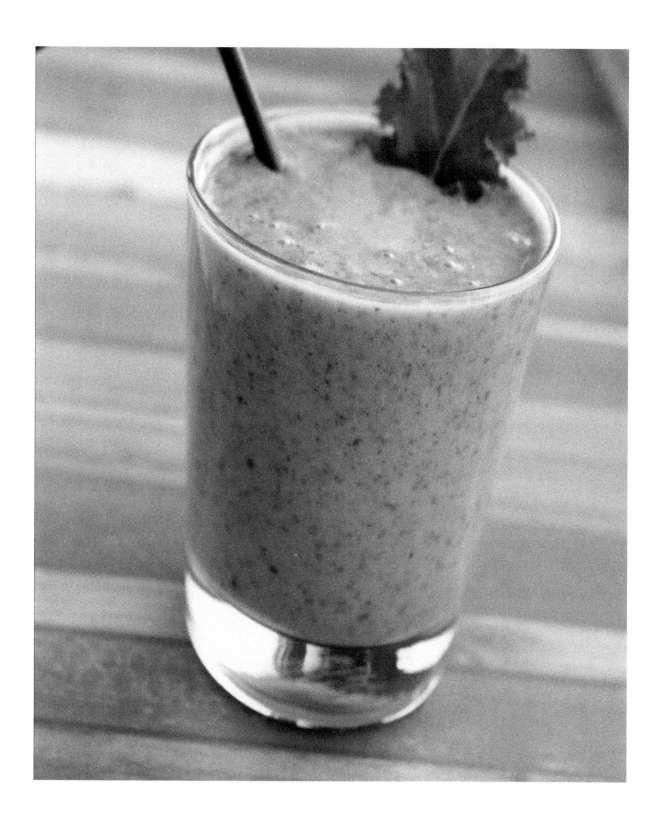

Sirtfood Wonder Smoothie

Amazing smoothie! So fresh and tasteful! It's perfect for breakfast!

Ingredients: 1 serving

- 1 cup arugula (rocket)
- 2 cups organic strawberries or blueberries
- 1 cup kale
- ½ teaspoon matcha green tea
- Juice of ½ lemon or lime
- 3 sprigs of parsley
- ½ cup of watercress
- ¾ cup of water

Directions:

- Add all the ingredients except matcha to a blender and whizz up until very smooth.
- Add the matcha green tea powder and give it a final blitz until well mixed.
- Enjoy!

Nutritional info per serving: Calories 145, Fat 2g, Carbohydrates 7g, Protein 3g

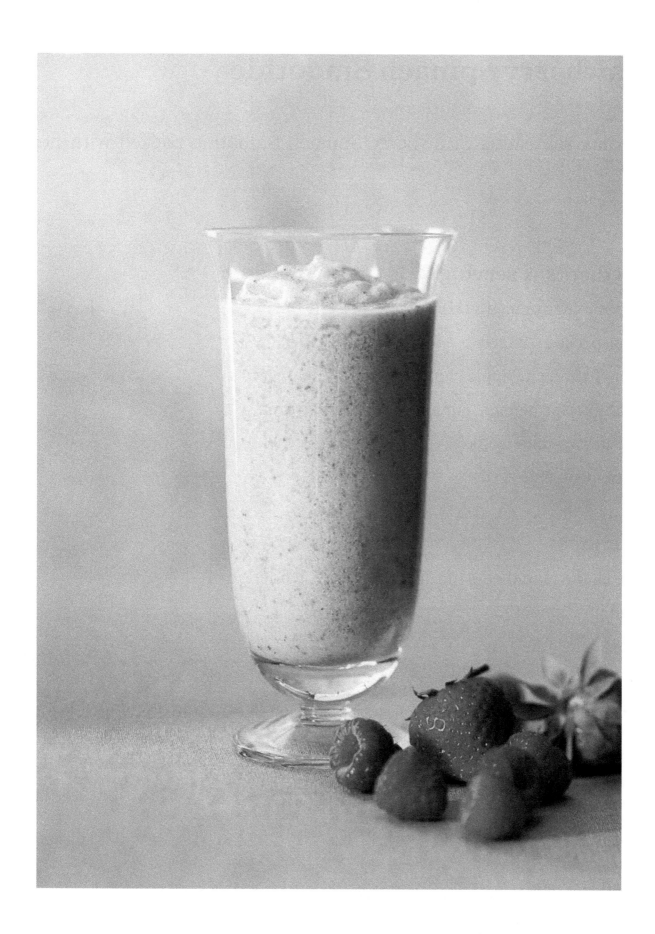

Strawberry Spinach Smoothie

A creamy refreshing Strawberry Spinach Smoothie packed with healthy ingredients!

Ingredients: 1 serving

- 1 cup whole frozen strawberries
- 3 cups packed spinach
- ¼ cup frozen pineapple chunks
- 1 medium ripe banana, cut into chunks and frozen
- 1 cup unsweetened milk
- 1 tablespoon chia seeds

Directions:

- Place all the ingredients in a high-powered blender.
- Blend until smooth.
- Enjoy!

Nutritional info per serving: Calories 266, Fat 8g, Carbohydrates 48g, Protein 9g

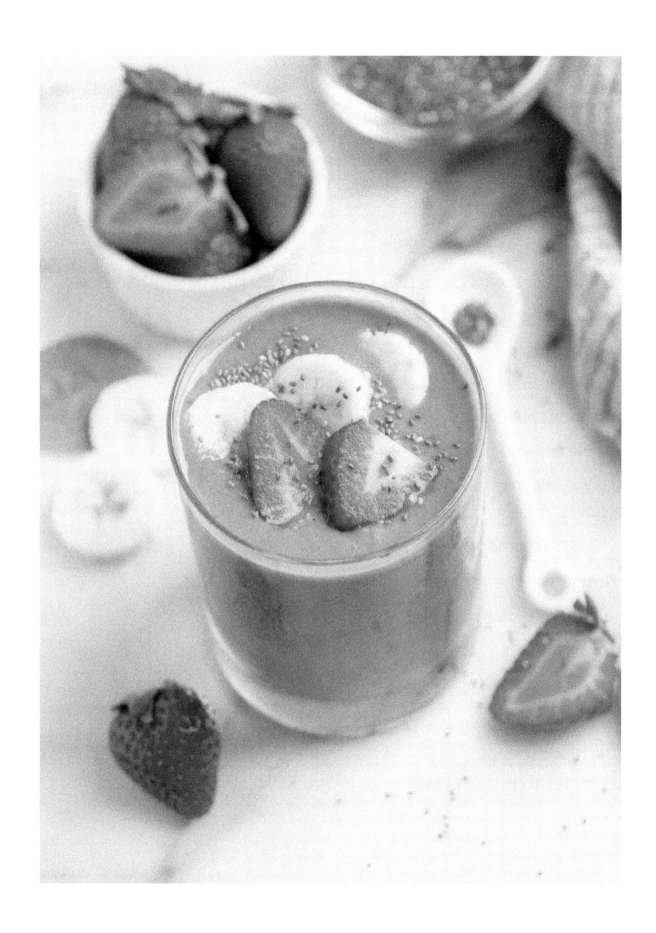

Berry Turmeric Smoothie

Berry Turmeric Smoothie with blueberries, spinach, ginger and honey. The perfect healthy breakfast smoothie to kick start your day!

Ingredients: 1 serving

- 1 ½ cups frozen mixed berries (blueberries, blackberries and raspberries)
- ½ teaspoon ground turmeric
- 2 cups baby spinach
- ¾ cup unsweetened vanilla almond milk, or milk of choice
- ½ cup non-fat plain Greek yogurt, or yoghurt of choice
- ¼ teaspoon ground ginger
- 2-3 teaspoons honey
- 3 tablespoons old-fashioned rolled oats

Directions:

- Place all the ingredients in a high-powered blender.
- Blend until smooth.
- Taste and adjust sweetness as desired.
- Enjoy immediately!

Nutritional info per serving: Calories 151, Fat 2g, Carbohydrates 27g, Protein 8g

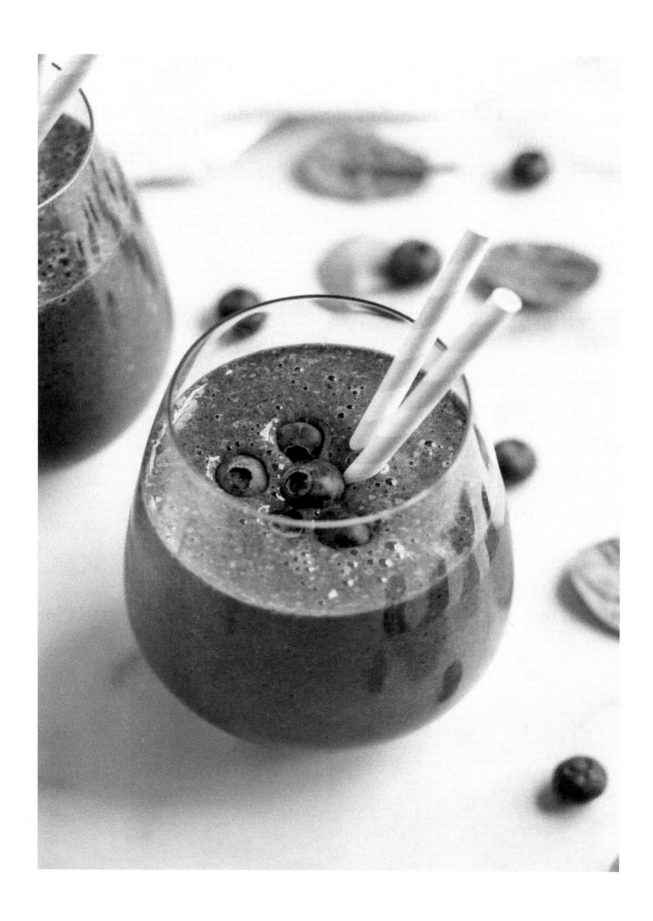

Mango Green Smoothie

A sweet, cream, and healthy Mango Green Smoothie that tastes like a tropical vacation!

Ingredients: 1 serving

- 1 ½ cups frozen mango pieces
- 1 cup packed baby spinach leaves
- 1 ripe banana
- ¾ cup unsweetened vanilla almond milk

Directions:

- Place all the ingredients in a blender.
- Blend until smooth.
- Enjoy!

Nutritional info per serving: Calories 229, Fat 2g, Carbohydrates 72g, Protein 2g

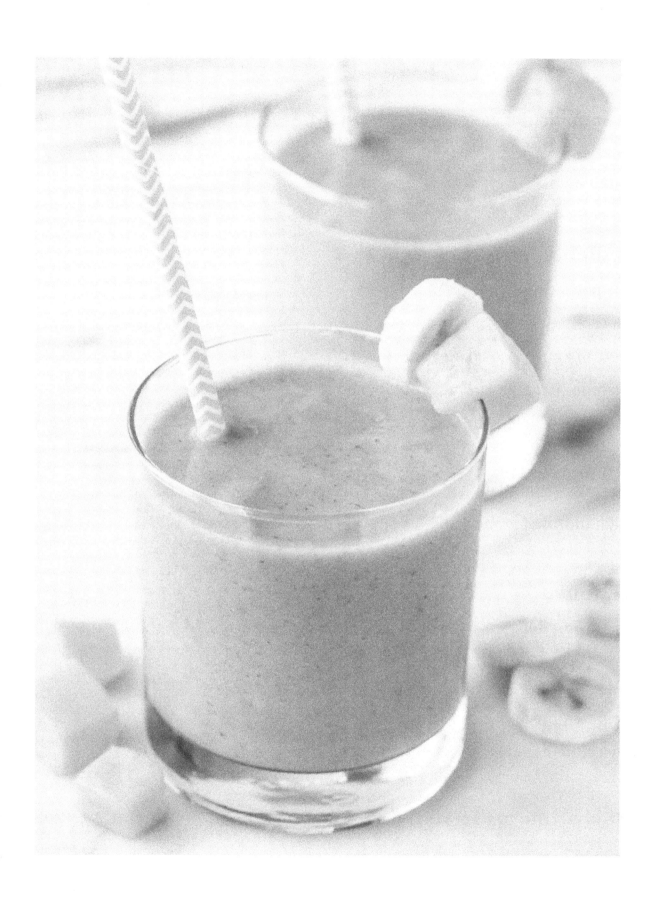

Apple Avocado Smoothie

A green apple avocado smoothie that tastes delicious! This is the perfect green smoothie for weight loss!

Ingredients: 1 serving

- 2 cups packed spinach
- ½ medium avocado
- 1 medium apple, peeled and quartered
- ½ medium banana, cut into chunks and frozen
- ½ cup unsweetened almond milk
- 1 teaspoon honey
- ¼ teaspoon ground ginger
- Small handful of ice cubes

Directions:

- In the ordered list, add the almond milk, spinach, avocado, banana, apples, honey, ginger, and ice to a high-powered blender.
- Blend until smooth.
- Taste and adjust sweetness and spices as desired.
- Enjoy immediately!

Nutritional info per serving: Calories 206, Fat 11g, Carbohydrates 15g, Protein 5g

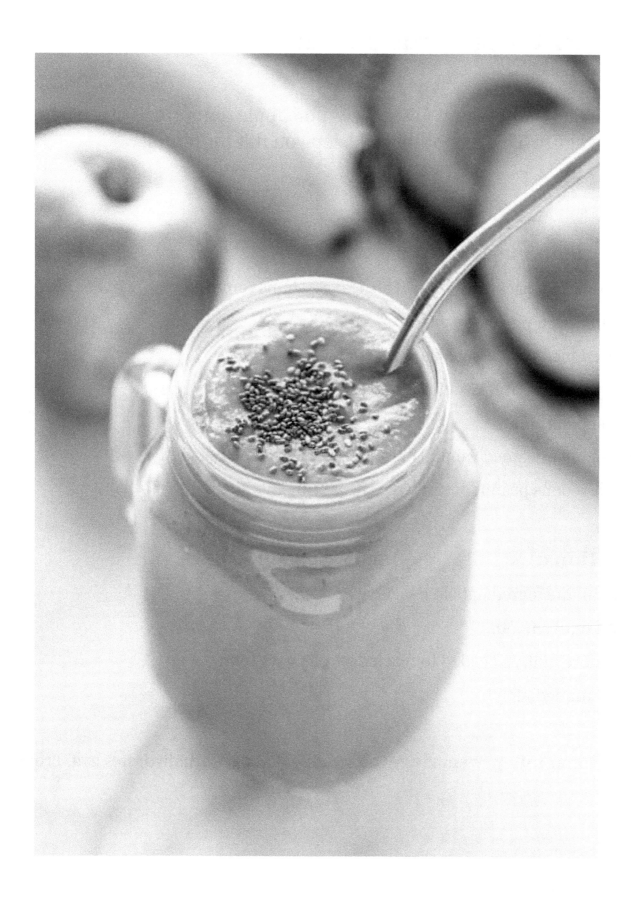

Kale Pineapple Smoothie

A delicious and creamy green kale pineapple smoothie with banana and Greek yogurt. This smoothie will keep you full for hours!

Ingredients: 1 serving

- 2 cups lightly packed chopped kale leaves, stems removed
- ¼ cup frozen pineapple pieces
- 1 frozen medium banana, cut into chunks
- ¼ cup non-fat Greek yogurt
- 2 teaspoons honey
- ¾ cup unsweetened vanilla almond milk, or any milk of choice
- 2 tablespoons peanut butter, creamy or crunchy

Directions:

- Place all the ingredients in a blender.
- Blend until smooth.
- Add more milk as needed to reach desired consistency.
- Enjoy immediately!

Nutritional info per serving: Calories 187, Fat 9g, Carbohydrates 27g, Protein 8g

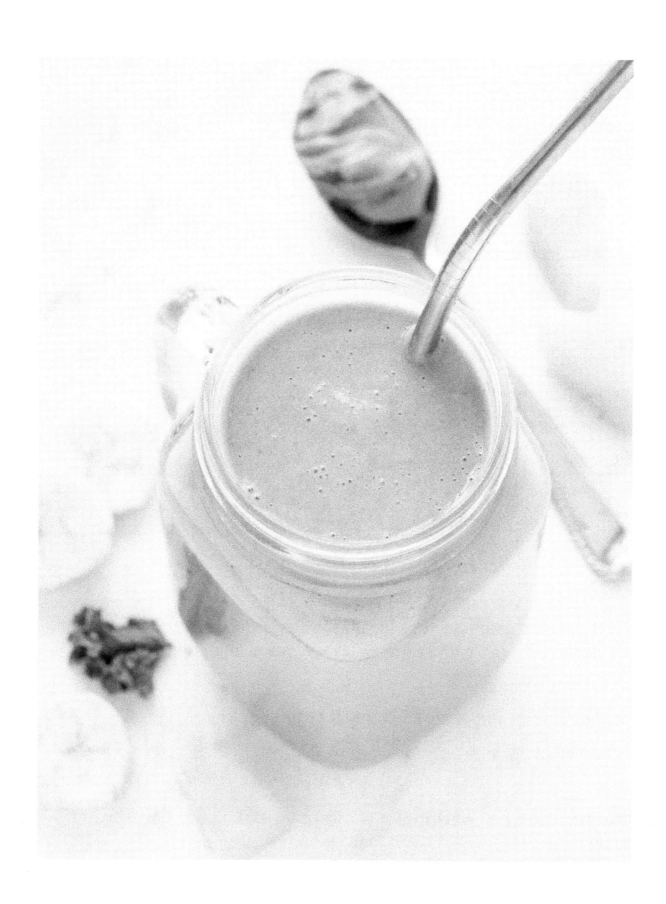

Blueberry Banana Avocado Smoothie

With antioxidants and healthy fats from spinach, avocado, and flax, this smoothie promotes glowing skin!

Ingredients: 1 serving

- 1 medium ripe banana, peeled
- 2 cups frozen blueberries
- 1 cup fresh spinach
- 1 tablespoon ground flaxseed meal
- ½ ripe avocado
- 1 tablespoon almond butter
- ¼ teaspoon cinnamon
- ½ cup unsweetened vanilla almond milk

Directions:

- Place all the ingredients in your blender in the ordered list: vanilla almond milk, spinach, banana, avocado, blueberries, flaxseed meal, and almond butter.
- Blend until smooth.
- If you like a thicker smoothie, add a small handful of ice.
- Enjoy immediately!

Nutritional info per serving: Calories 298, Fat 14.4g, Carbohydrates 38.1g, Protein 8g

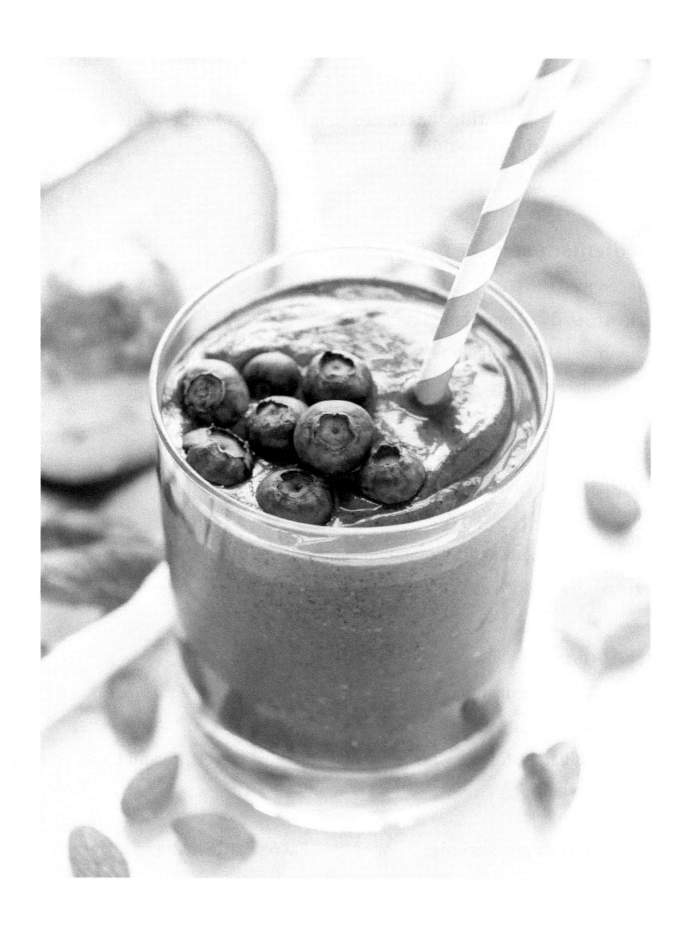

Carrot Smoothie

A healthy carrot smoothie that tastes just like carrot cake! This smoothie is made with banana, pineapple, and carrot cake spices!

Ingredients: 1 serving

- 1 cup chopped carrots
- ¼ cup frozen diced pineapple
- ½ cup frozen sliced banana
- ¼ teaspoon cinnamon
- 1 tablespoon flaked coconut
- ½ cup Greek yogurt
- 2 tablespoons toasted walnuts
- Pinch nutmeg
- ½ cup unsweetened vanilla almond milk, or milk of choice
- For topping: shredded carrots, coconut, crushed walnuts

Directions:

- Add all the ingredients into a blender.
- Blend until smooth.
- Enjoy immediately, topped with additional shredded carrots, coconut, and crushed walnuts as desired!

Nutritional info per serving: Calories 279, Fat 6g, Carbohydrates 48g, Protein 7g

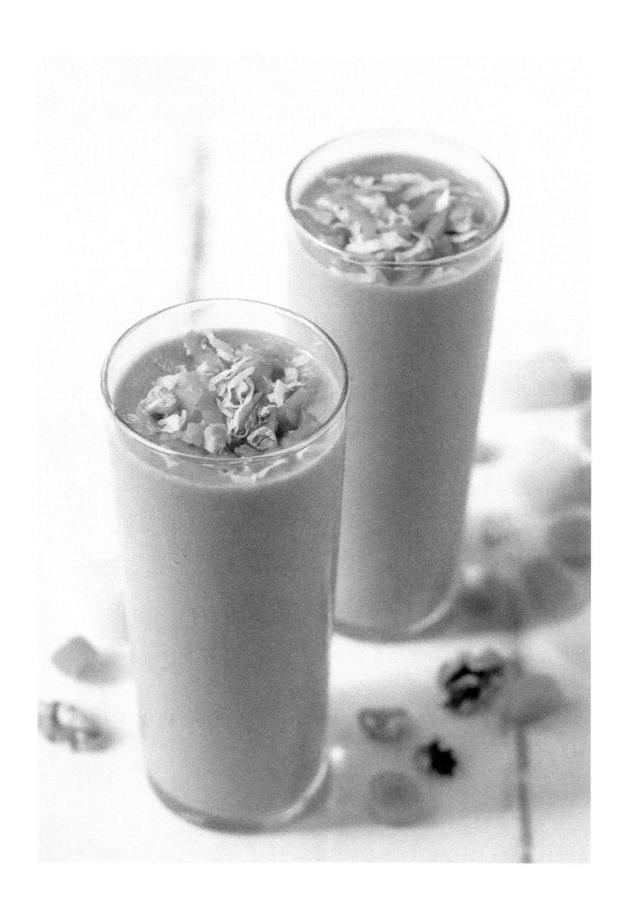

Matcha Berry Smoothie

This glowing Matcha Berry Smoothie is made with green tea powder, berries and all natural plant-based ingredients!

Ingredients: 1 serving

- ½ banana
- ½-tablespoon matcha powder
- 1 cup almond milk
- 1 cup frozen blueberries
- ¼ teaspoon ground ginger
- ½ tablespoon chia seeds
- ¼ teaspoon ground cinnamon

Directions:

- In a blender, blend the almond milk, banana, blueberries, matcha powder, chia seeds, cinnamon, and ginger until smooth.
- Enjoy immediately!

Nutritional info per serving: Calories 212, Fat 5g, Carbohydrates 34g, Protein 8g

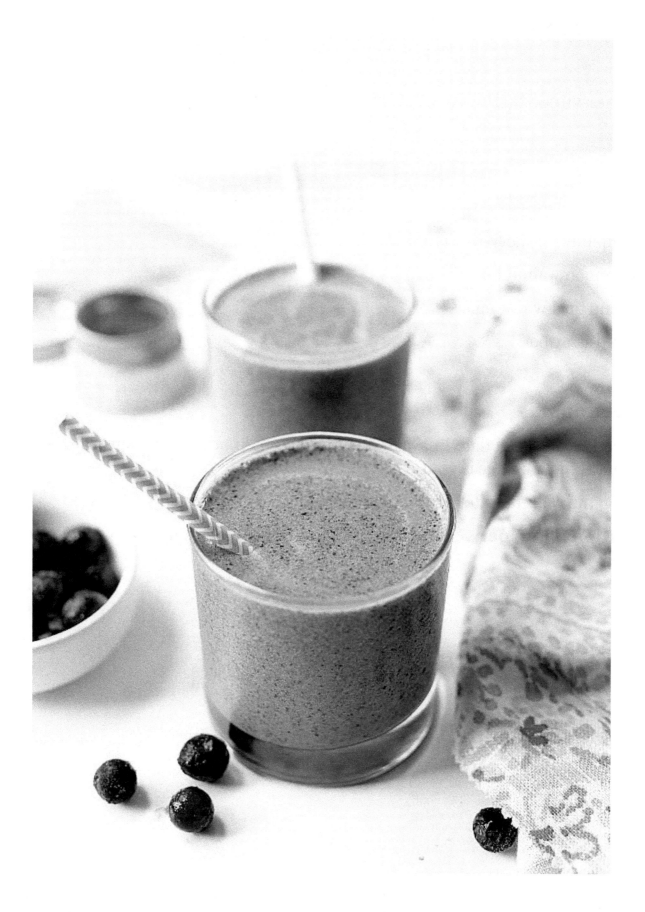

Date & Walnut Porridge

Another super tasty way to start your day!

Ingredients: 1 serving

- 1 Medjool date
- ¾ cup milk or dairy-free alternative
- 1 teaspoon walnut butter
- 1/3 cup buckwheat flakes
- ½ cup strawberries

Directions:

- Place the milk and date in a pan, heat gently, then add the buckwheat flakes and cook until the porridge is your desired consistency.
- Stir in the walnut butter or walnuts, top with the strawberries and enjoy!

Nutritional info per serving: Calories 212, Fat 14g Carbohydrates 29g, Protein 8g

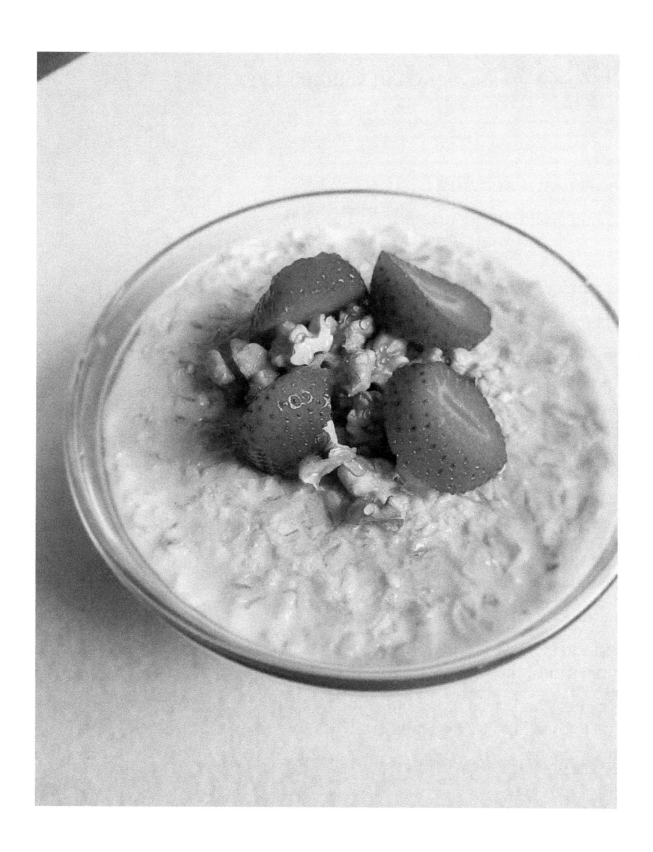

Sirtfood Breakfast Scramble

So delicious! A great way to start your morning!

Ingredients: 1 serving

- 1 teaspoon ground turmeric
- 2 eggs
- 1/3 oz parsley, finely chopped
- 1 teaspoon mild curry powder
- ¼ cup kale, roughly chopped
- 1 handful of button mushrooms, thinly sliced
- 1 teaspoon extra virgin olive oil
- ½ bird's eye chili, thinly sliced

Directions:

- Mix the turmeric and curry powder and add a little water until you have reached a light paste.
- Steam the kale for 2-3 minutes.
- Heat the oil in a frying pan over a medium heat and fry the chili and mushrooms for 2-3 minutes until they have started to brown and soften.
- Add the eggs and spice paste and cook over a medium heat, then add the kale and continue to cook for a further minute.
- Finally, add the parsley, mix well and enjoy!

Nutritional info per serving: Calories 268, Fat 21g, Carbohydrates 13g, Protein 10g

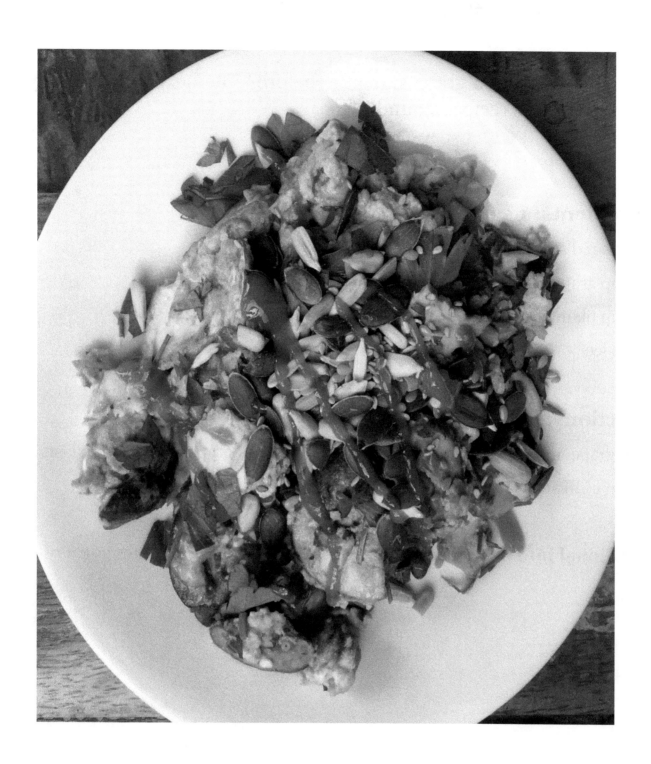

Simple Grape Smoothie

Have you ever had a grape smoothie before? The next time you buy red grapes, keep this recipe in mind!

Ingredients: 1 serving

- 2 cups red seedless grapes
- ¼ cup grape juice
- ½ cup plain yogurt
- 1 cup ice

Directions:

- Add grape juice to the blender. Then add yogurt and grapes. Add the ice last.
- Blend until smooth and enjoy!

Nutritional info per serving: Calories 161, Fat 4g, Carbohydrates 39g, Protein 2g

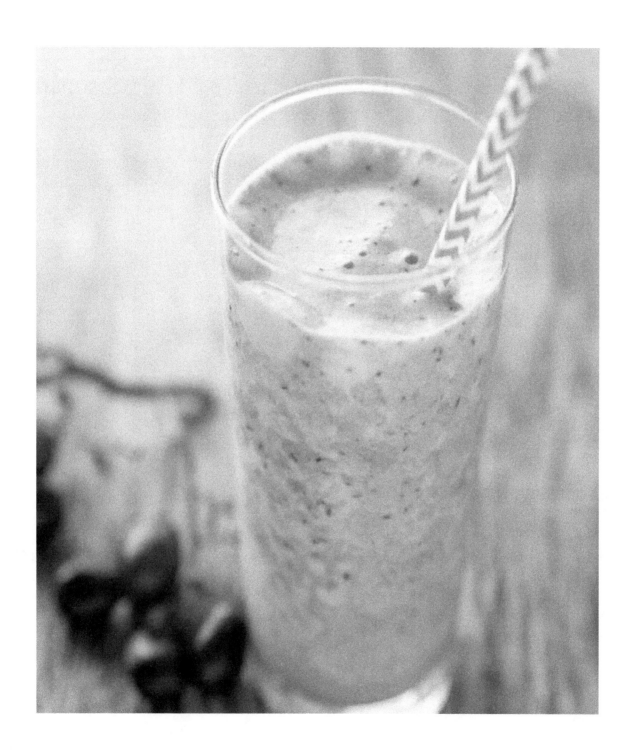

Ginger Plum Smoothie

When it comes to fruit smoothies, plums may not be the first flavor you think of, but trust me, this is a very sweet and tasty drink!

Ingredients: 1 serving

- 1 ripe plum, fresh or frozen, pitted but not peeled
- ½ cup plain yogurt
- ½ cup orange juice, or other fruit juice
- 1 teaspoon grated fresh ginger

Directions:

- Put all the ingredients in a blender and blend until smooth.
- Serve immediately and enjoy!

Nutritional info per serving: Calories 124, Fat 2g, Carbohydrates 26g, Protein 3g

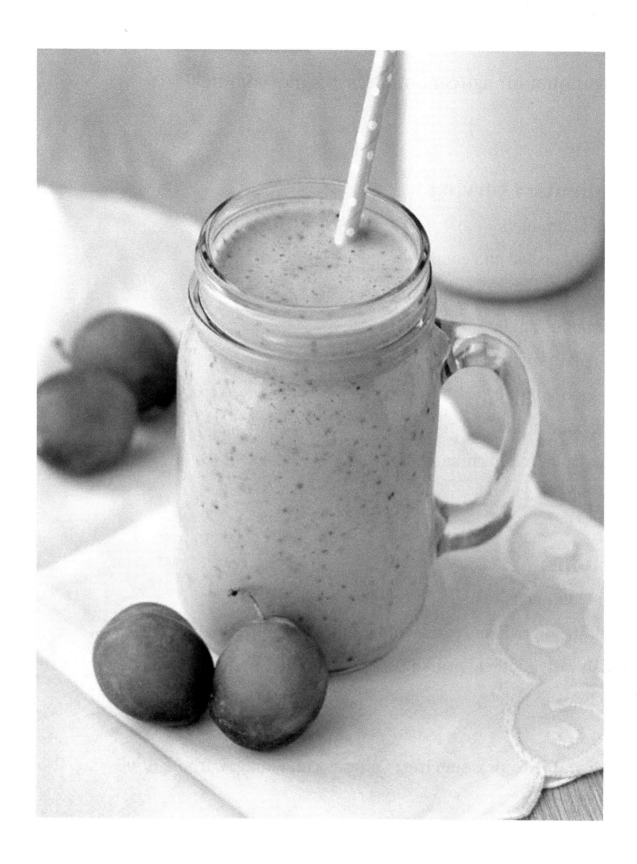

Kumquat Mango Smoothie

This Kumquat Mango Smoothie tastes like summer!

Ingredients: 1 serving

- 15 small kumquats
- ½ mango, peeled and chopped
- ¾ cup unsweetened almond milk
- ¼ teaspoon vanilla
- ½ cup plain yogurt
- ¼ teaspoon nutmeg
- 1 tablespoon honey
- ½ teaspoon ground cinnamon
- 5 ice cubes

Directions:

- Cut the kumquats in half and remove any seeds.
- Add all the ingredients to a blender and blend until smooth.
- Garnish with another sprinkling of cinnamon, if desired.
- Enjoy immediately!

Nutritional info per serving: Calories 116, Fat 2g, Carbohydrates 22g, Protein 5g

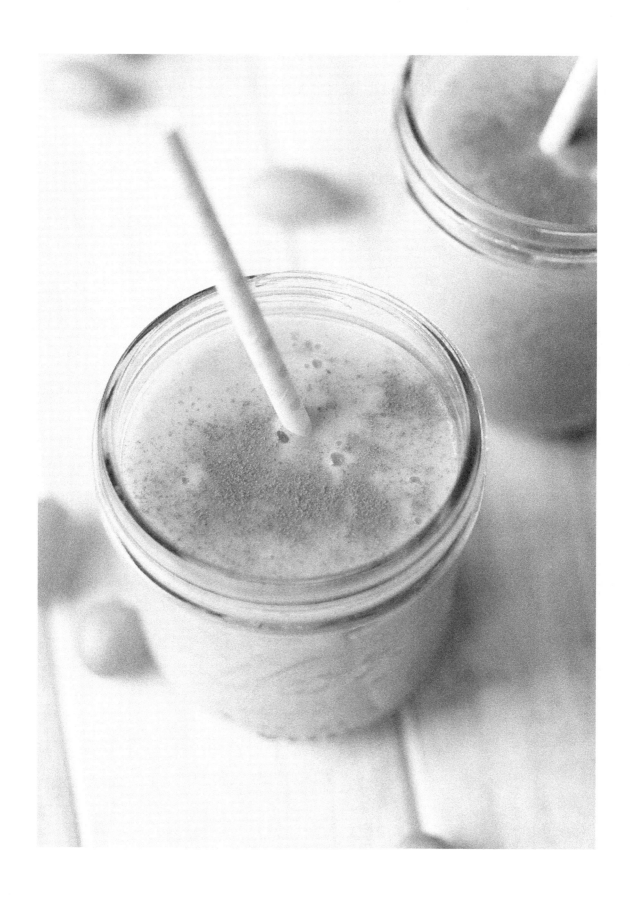

Cranberry Smoothie

Easy to make, with lots of healthy ingredients, this cranberry smoothie is tasty and refreshing!

Ingredients: 1 serving

- ½ cup frozen cranberries
- ½ banana
- ¼ cup orange juice
- ¼ cup frozen blueberries
- ¼ cup low fat Greek yogurt

Directions:

- Add all the ingredients to a blender and blend until smooth. Add a little more orange juice if you prefer it a little thinner. Enjoy immediately!

Nutritional info per serving: Calories 165, Fat 1g, Carbohydrates 31g, Protein 8g

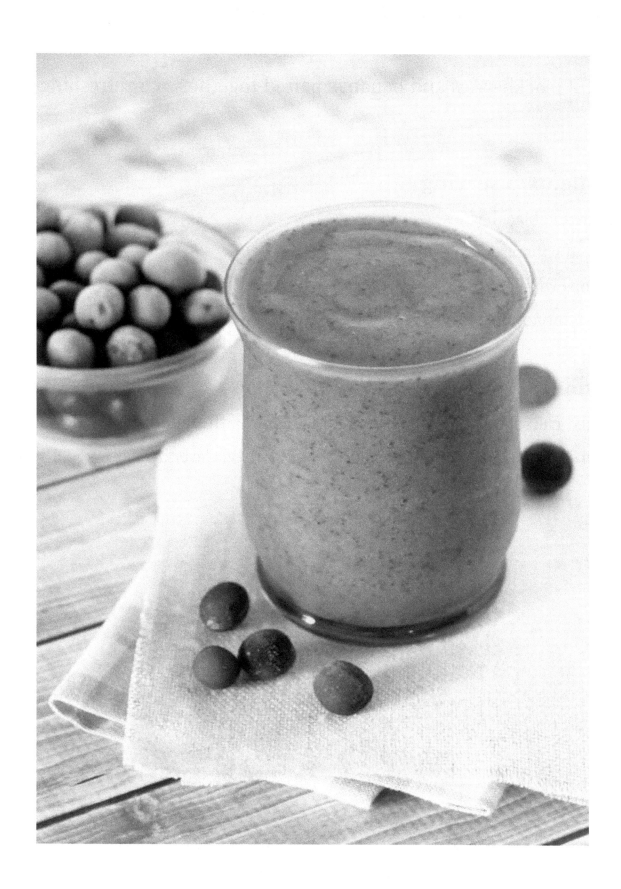

Blackberry Banana Smoothie

Flavorful blackberries and bananas paired together in a refreshing frozen drink!

Ingredients: 1 serving

- 1 cup frozen blackberries
- ½ frozen banana
- 2-3 drops vanilla
- ½ cup almond milk, or milk of choice

Directions:

- Put milk, fruit and vanilla in a blender and blend until smooth. Enjoy!

Nutritional info per serving: Calories 208, Fat 2g, Carbohydrates 36g, Protein 5g

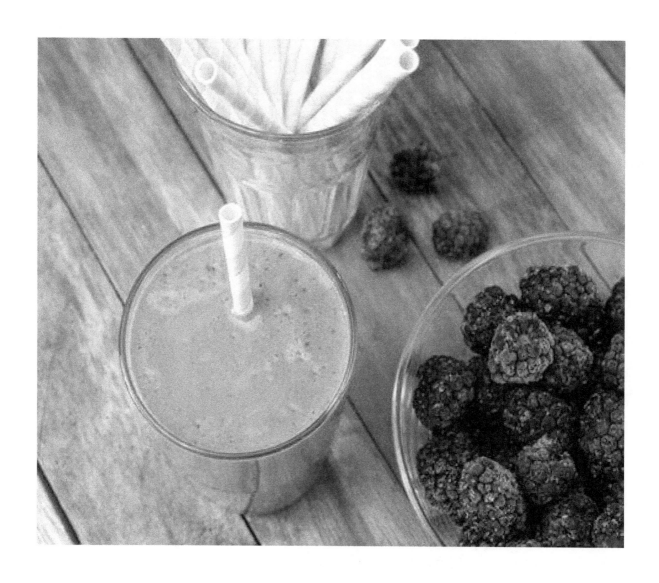

Creamy Pineapple Cucumber Smoothie

A creamy, 6-ingredient cucumber smoothie with coconut, pineapple, lime and greens!

Ingredients: 1 serving

- 1 cup cubed pineapple
- ½ cup sliced cucumber
- ¼ cup coconut milk
- 1 large handful greens, spinach or kale
- 1 medium lime, zested and juiced
- ½ large ripe banana, peeled
- ½ cup water
- 2-4 ice cubes

Directions:

- Add cucumber, pineapple, frozen banana, lime zest, coconut milk, water, lime juice, greens, and ice cubes to a blender and blend until smooth and creamy.
- For a thicker smoothie, add more ice. For a thinner smoothie, add more liquid of choice.
- Enjoy immediately!

Nutritional info per serving: Calories 215, Fat 3g, Carbohydrates 46g, Protein 6g

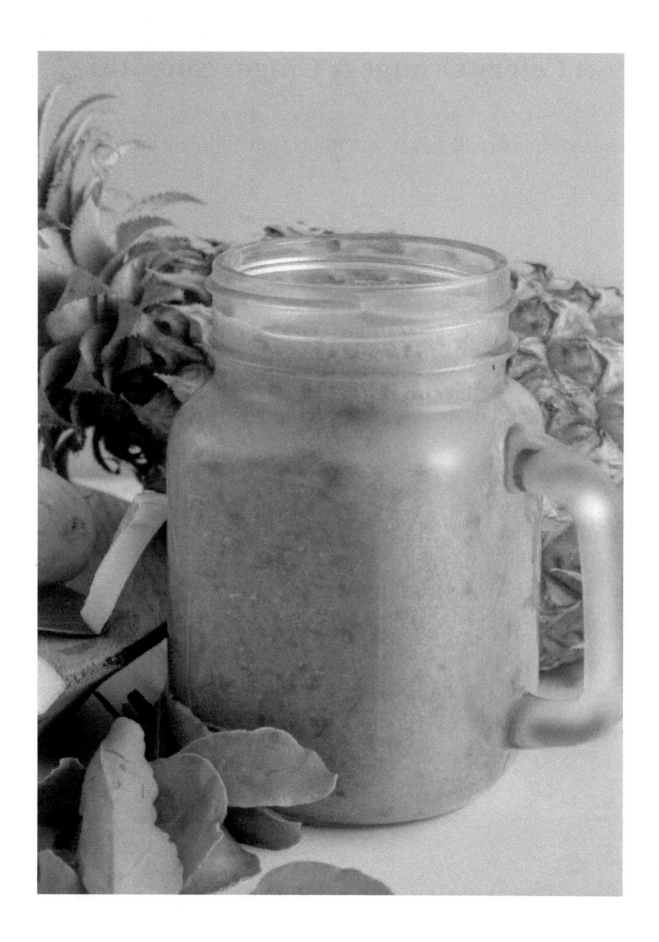

Carrot Celery Orange & Ginger Smoothie

This fruit, vegetable and ginger smoothie is not only delicious, but it's super healthy too!

Ingredients: 1 serving

- 1 carrot
- 1 orange
- 1 slice ginger
- ½ stick celery
- 1 cup ice

Directions:

- Put all the ingredients to a blender.
- Blend until desired consistency is reached.
- Enjoy immediately.

Nutritional info per serving: Calories 234, Fat 1g, Carbohydrates 52g, Protein 9g

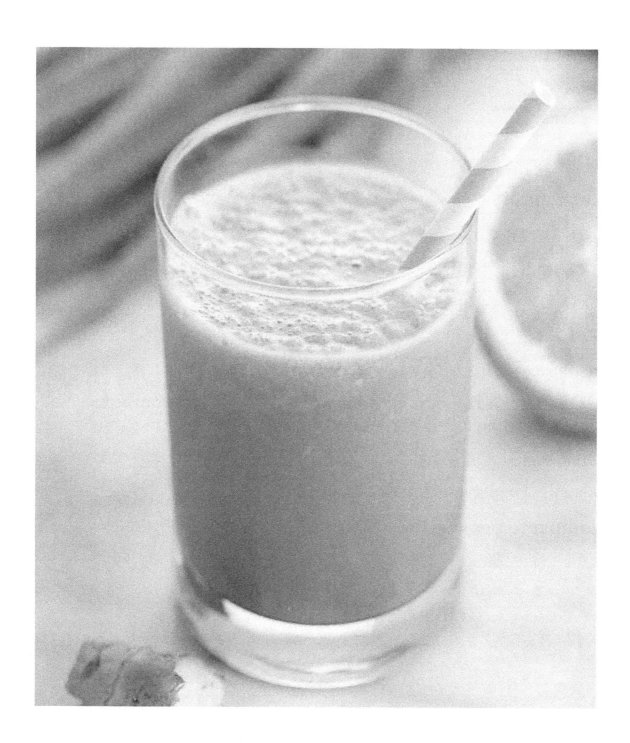

Strawberry Orange Juice

Brighten your morning with a shot of strawberries in your orange juice!

Ingredients: 2 servings

- 12 strawberries
- 6 oranges
- ½ teaspoon vanilla extract

Directions:

- Remove the leaves from the strawberries.
- Cut the oranges in half and juice them. Place the juice, strawberries and vanilla extract in a blender and blend until smooth.
- Enjoy immediately!

Nutritional info per serving: Calories 338, Fat 4g, Carbohydrates 91g, Protein 9g

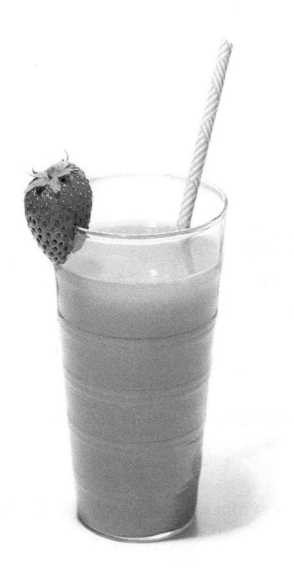

Tropical Watercress Juice

This Tropical Watercress Juice is packed with watercress and tropical fruits!

Ingredients: 1 serving

- ½ cup orange juice
- ½ cup watercress
- ½ teaspoon vanilla extract
- ½ banana, chopped and frozen
- ¼ cup chopped pineapple
- ¼ cup chopped mango

Directions:

- Blend watercress and juice until smooth, then add the rest of the ingredients. Blend until smooth and enjoy!

Nutritional info per serving: Calories 184, Fat 1g, Carbohydrates 41g, Protein 4g

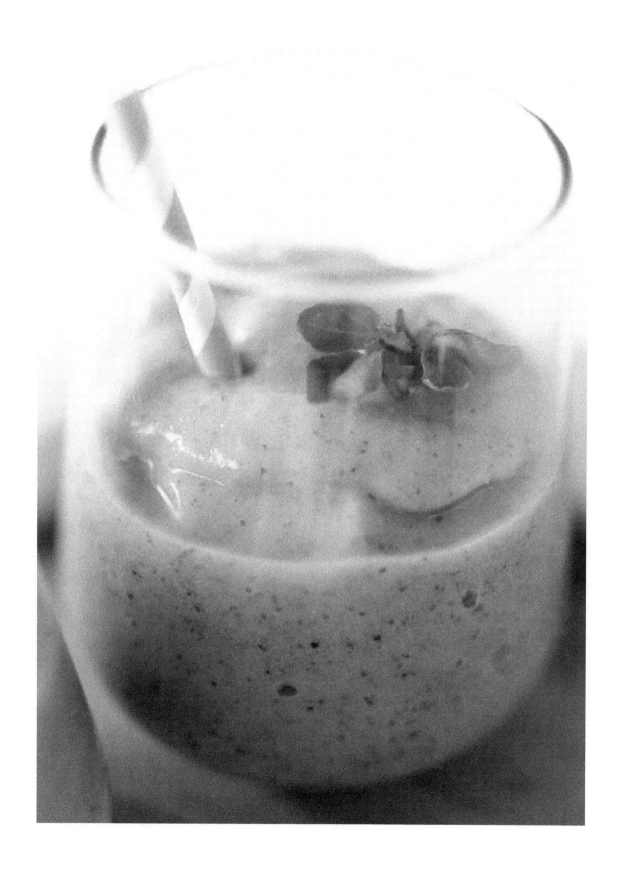

Arugula Apple Smoothie

This tasty Arugula Apple Smoothie is packed with sweet apples and mango, creamy Greek yogurt, and peppery arugula!

Ingredients: 1 serving

- ½ cup arugula
- 1 medium apple, peeled and chopped
- 2/3 cup frozen mango
- ½ lemon juiced
- ½ cup plain non-fat Greek yogurt
- 2/3 cup water

Ingredients:

- Put all the ingredients in a blender.
- Blend until smooth.
- Enjoy immediately!

Nutritional info per serving: Calories 231, Fat 1g, Carbohydrates 43g, Protein 12g

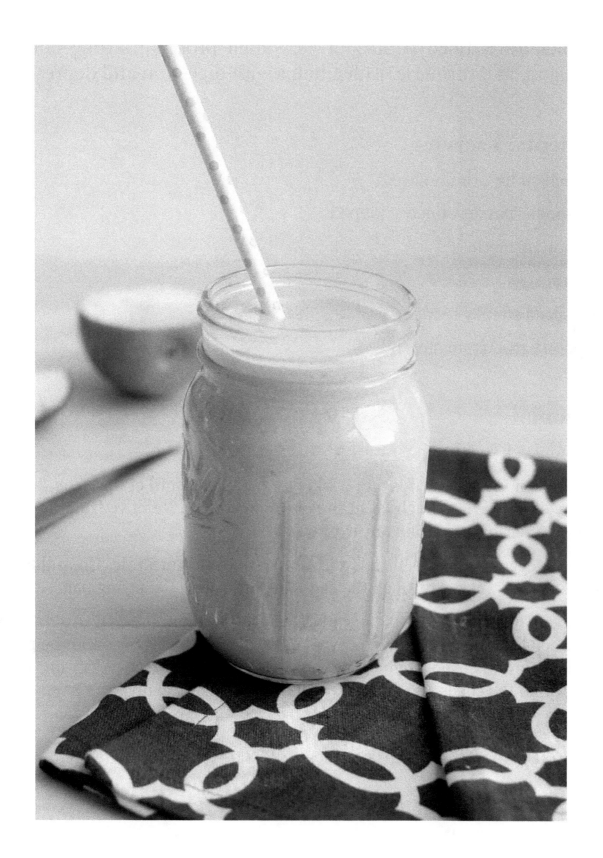

Sirtfood Omelette

This Omelette is filled with endives, which promote strong bones and better vision, and turmeric, which helps with digestion and depression!

Ingredients: 1 serving

- ¼ cup red endive, thinly sliced
- 2 tablespoons parsley, finely chopped
- 1 teaspoon turmeric
- 2 medium eggs
- ½ cup sliced streaky bacon
- 1 teaspoon extra virgin olive oil

Directions:

- Heat a nonstick frying pan.

- Cut the bacon into thin strips and cook over high heat until crispy. You don't need to add any oil, there is enough fat in the bacon to cook it. Remove from the pan and place on a paper towel to drain any excess fat.

- Whisk the eggs and mix with the endive, parsley and turmeric. Chop the cooked bacon into cubes and stir through the eggs. Heat the oil in the frying pan.

- Add the egg mixture and, using a spatula, move it around the pan to start cooking the egg. Keep the cooked egg bits moving and swirl the raw egg around the pan until the omelette level is even. Reduce the heat and let the omelette firm up. Ease the spatula around the edges and fold the omelette in half or roll up and serve.

Nutritional info per serving: Calories 221, Fat 9g, Carbohydrates 4g, Protein 12g

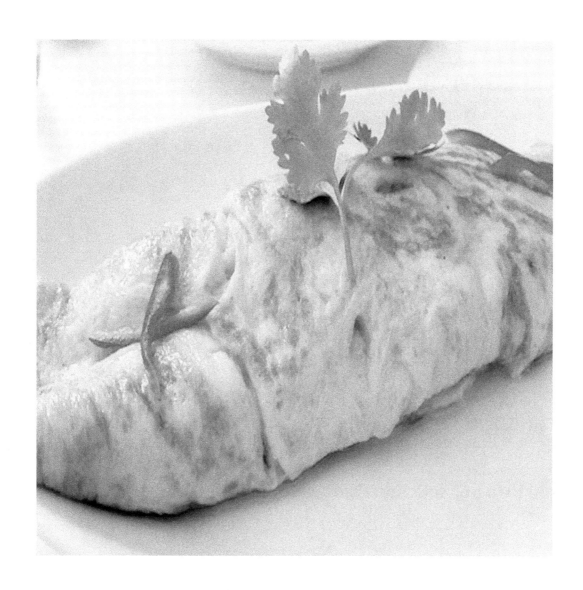

Sirtfood Chocolate Strawberry Milk

The Sirtfood Chocolate Strawberry Milk is one of the most delicious way to start your day!

Ingredients: 1 serving

- 1 cup strawberries, hulled and halved
- ½ oz pitted Medjool dates
- 1 tablespoon cocoa powder
- ½ oz walnuts
- 1 cup milk, or dairy-free alternative

Directions:

- Place all the ingredients in a blender.
- Blend until smooth
- Enjoy immediately!

Nutritional info per serving: Calories 202, Fat 1g, Carbohydrates 23g, Protein 11g

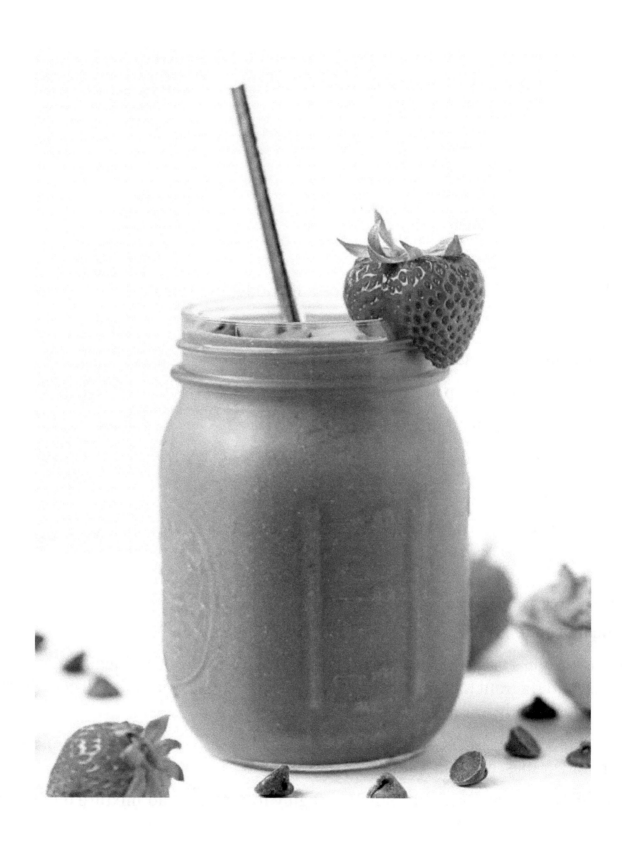

Cranberry & Orange Granola

Candied orange peel is the star of this granola!

Ingredients: 2 cups

- 2 tablespoons dried cranberries
- 2 tablespoons candied orange peel, sliced into long thin stripes
- ½ cup sliced almonds
- 1 cup old fashioned oats
- ¼ cup pure maple syrup
- ½ tablespoon unsalted butter, melted
- ½ teaspoon grapeseed oil
- 2 tablespoons golden raisins
- Nonstick vegetable oil spray

Directions:

- Preheat oven to 300° F.
- Spread oats on a large rimmed baking sheet. Toast, stirring occasionally, until lightly browned and fragrant (about 20 minutes). Transfer to a heatproof bowl; add almonds and let cool slightly.
- Coat some baking sheet with non stick vegetable oil spray. Whisk maple syrup, butter, and grapeseed oil in a small bowl to blend.
- Pour syrup mixture over oats; stir thoroughly to coat. Spread mixture on prepared sheet.
- Bake granola, stirring occasionally, until the oats are light golden (about 15 minutes). Stir in the cranberries and raisins; bake for 10 minutes longer.

- Remove granola from oven and let cool slightly. Stir in the orange peel.
- Let cool completely, then break into pieces and enjoy immediately!

Nutritional info per serving: Calories 118, Fat 4.3, Carbohydrates 18.7g, Protein 2.7g

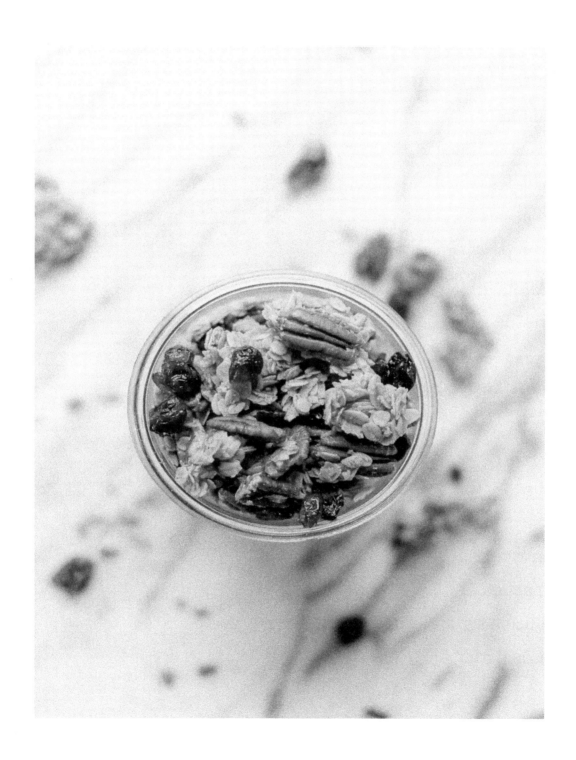

Creamy Coconut Porridge

This Creamy Coconut Porridge can be served warm or chilled! Top with your favourite seasonal fruit and a drizzle of maple syrup!

Ingredients: 2 servings

- ¼ cup walnuts
- ½ cup Kasha (Roasted Buckwheat Kernels)
- 2 Medjool dates, pitted
- 1 tablespoon chia seeds
- 1 tablespoon pure maple syrup
- 1 cup coconut milk
- Pinch of salt

Options for the Toppings:

- Mango
- Banana
- Cocoa Nibs
- Unsweetened, toasted coconut
- Cinnamon
- Macadamia nuts
- Drizzle of maplt syrup
- Other seasonal fruit

Directions:

• In a large glass jar, soak the kasha and walnuts overnight, or at least 4 hours.

• Rinse the kasha and walnuts through a fine mesh strainer under running water, shaking the strainer several times ensure through rinsing.

• Place all the ingredients in a blender and blend for abut 20 seconds. Scrape down sides and blend again for another 5-10 seconds.

• Can be served chilled or gently warmed. Top with favourite toppings, and enjoy!

Nutritional info per serving: Calories 420, Fat 28g, Carbohydrates 57g, Protein 12g

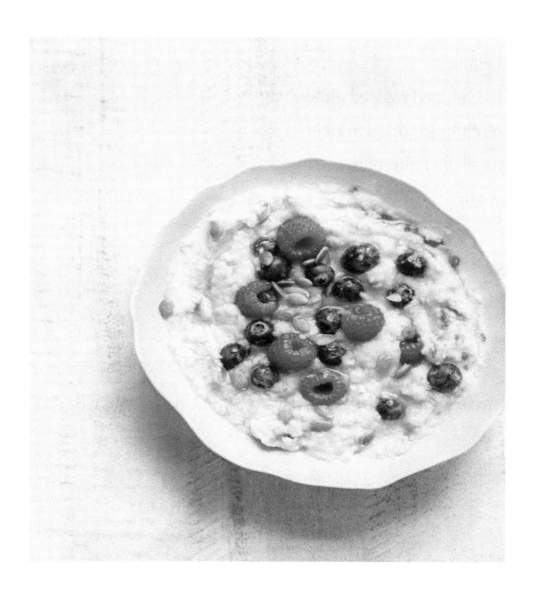

Homemade Muesli

This Homemade Muesli is so easy to prepare! A good way to start your day!

Ingredients: 2 cups

- ½ cup barley flakes
- 2 tablespoons dried blueberries or chopped dates
- ½ cup rye flakes
- 1 cup old fashioned oats
- ¼ cup flaxseed meal
- 2 tablespoons chopped roasted almonds
- 2 tablespoons chopped dried apricots
- 2 tablespoons shelled pumpkin seeds
- 1/8 teaspoon salt

Directions:

- Mix all the ingredients in a bowl.
- Enjoy!

Nutritional info per serving: Calories 250, Fat 8g, Carbohydrates 36g, Protein 10.5g

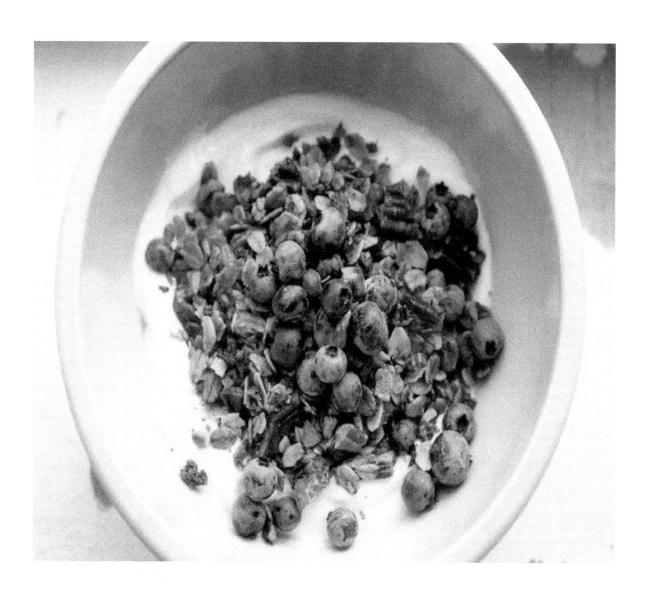

Fresh Herbs and Cheese Scramble

This no-fuss scramble recipe is easy to adjust to fit your tastes! So flavorful!

Ingredients: 2 servings

- 3 eggs
- ½ green onion, finely chopped
- ½ teaspoon fresh chopped cilantro
- ½ teaspoon fresh chopped chives
- 1 tablespoon milk
- 1/8 cup shredded cheese
- Salt and pepper to taste

Directions:

- Beat the eggs with milk until frothy.
- Prepare a large skillet by setting to medium heat and spraying generously with cooking spray.
- Add the eggs to the hot skillet and sprinkle fresh herbs over the eggs. Season with salt and pepper to taste.
- As soon as the eggs begin to set, start to scramble, gradually adding the cheese.
- Cook until completely set. Garnish with an additional sprinkle of fresh herbs if desired. Enjoy!

Nutritional info per serving: Calories 274, Fat 18g, Carbohydrates 7g, Protein 16g

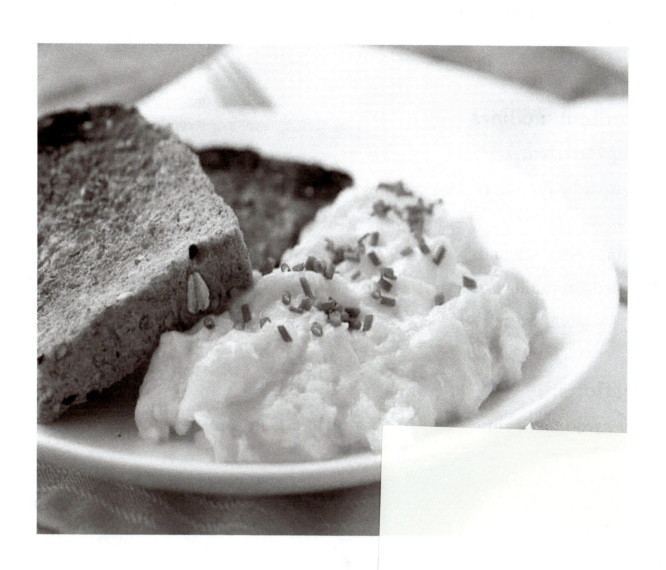

Dark Chocolate Almond Bars

Easy to prepare! 6-ingredient Dark Chocolate Bars made from scratch and topped with toasted almonds!

Ingredients: 6 bars

- ½ cup cacao butter
- ½ cup cacao powder or unsweetened cocoa powder
- ¼ cup maple syrup
- ¼ cup roasted almonds
- ½ teaspoon vanilla extract
- 0.05 teaspoon sea salt

Directions:

- Melt cacao butter in a double boiler or in a glass mixing bowl set over a small saucepan with 1 inch of water over medium heat.

- Once melted, remove from heat and add maple syrup and whisk to combine. When the mixture is completely fluid with no separation, add cacao or cocoa powder and vanilla extract.

- Taste and adjust sweetness if needed.

Pour the chocolate into candy molds (if you have them), mini paper cupcake liners, or simply line a baking sheet with parchment paper and pour the chocolate on top. Top with roasted almonds and sprinkle of salt.

- Set in the refrigerator or freezer to harden for 30 minutes to 1 hour.

- Once completely solid, break or cut into pieces/bars. Enjoy!

Nutritional info per serving: Calories 239, Fat 18.5g, Carbohydrates 11.2g, Protein 2.8

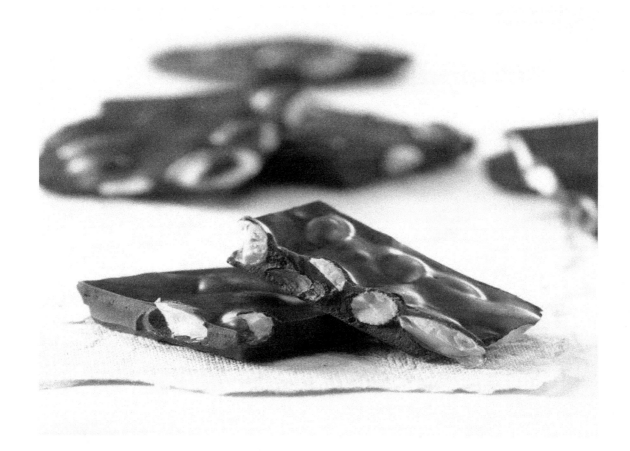

Coconut Yogurt Waffles

So simple to make! These gluten-free yogurt waffles are crisp on the outside and tender on the inside!

Ingredients: 4 waffles

- ½ cup dairy-free yogurt
- 2 tablespoons melted coconut oil or olive oil
- 1 cup unsweetened almond milk
- 1 ½ tablespoons maple syrup
- 1 ½ tablespoons coconut sugar or organic cane sugar
- 0.2 teaspoons salt
- 1 teaspoon baking powder
- ½ cup gluten-free rolled oats
- 1 ½ cups gluten-free flour blend
- ¾ teaspoon lemon juice or apple cider vinegar
- ¾ teaspoon pure vanilla extract (optional)

Optional Toppings

- Sliced banana, fresh fruit, coconut whipped cream, dairy-free yogurt

Directions:

- Combine almond milk and lemon juice or vinegar in a medium-size mixing bowl and let set for 5 minutes. Then add yogurt, coconut oil, vanilla extract, maple syrup and whisk thoroughly to combine. Set aside.
- Add dry ingredients to a large mixing bowl and whisk until well combined.

- Add wet ingredients to dry and mix until well incorporated. Let set for 10 minutes while your waffle iron preheats.

- Once waffle iron is ready, coat with non-stick spray or coconut oil and pour on about ½ cup of batter. Cook according to manufacturer instructions and then remove and place on a cooling rack set on a baking sheet in a 200° F oven to keep warm. Do not stack and keep them in a single layer to ensure crispiness.

- Serve immediately with desired toppings!

Nutritional info per serving: Calories 331, Fat 11.8g, Carbohydrates 49g, Protein 6.4g

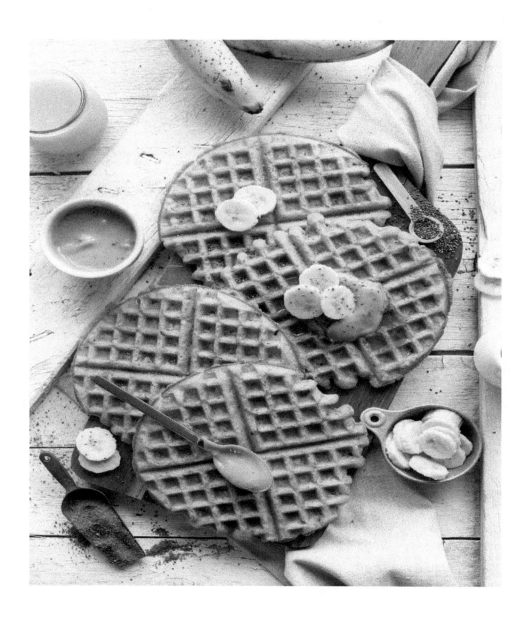

Cinnamon Buckwheat Bowls

Buckwheat is a great alternative to your breakfast oatmeal. It has a chewy and heartier texture!

Ingredients: 1 serving

- ½ cup buckwheat groats, rinsed
- ½ cup almond milk, or milk of choice
- ½ teaspoon cinnamon
- ½ cup water
- ½ teaspoon vanilla
- honey to serve
- sliced fruit to serve

Directions:

- In a small pot, add rinsed buckwheat groats, water, almond milk, cinnamon, and vanilla. Bring to a boil, then reduce to a simmer and cover with a lid. Simmer for 10 minutes.

- Turn off heat and let it steam, covered, for an additional 5 minutes.

- Fluff with a fork and portion into a bowl. Top with sliced fruit, a splash more milk, and a drizzle of honey, if desired.

Nutritional info per serving: Calories 182, Fat 1g, Carbohydrates 34g, Protein 6.7g

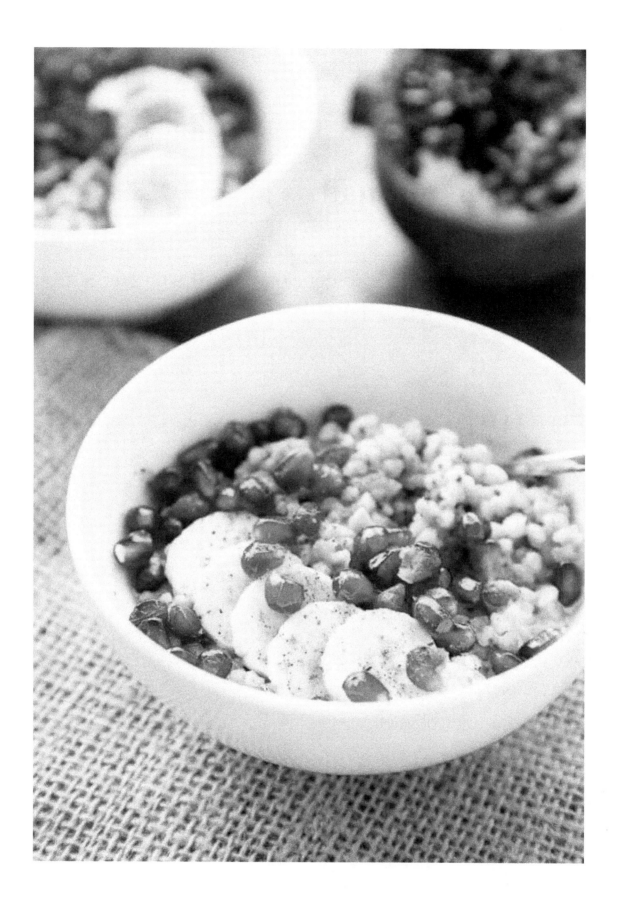

Light Bites

Sirtfood Salmon Salad

This Sirtfood Salmon Salad is so delicious! It's the perfect Sirtfood light bite!

Ingredients: 1 serving

- 1 cup rocket
- 2 oz chicory leaves
- 1 tablespoon capers
- 3 oz avocado, peeled, stoned and sliced
- 3,5 oz smoked salmon slices
- 1/8 cup walnuts, chopped
- 1 large Medjool date, pitted and chopped
- Juice of ¼ lemon
- 1 tablespoon extra virgin olive oil
- 3/8 cup parsley, chopped
- ½ oz celery leaves
- ¼ cup red onion, sliced

Directions:

• Place the salad leaves on a plate or in a large bowl. Mix all the remaining ingredients together and serve on top of the leaves.

Nutritional info per serving: Calories 194, Fat 9g, Carbohydrates 4.5g, Protein 21g

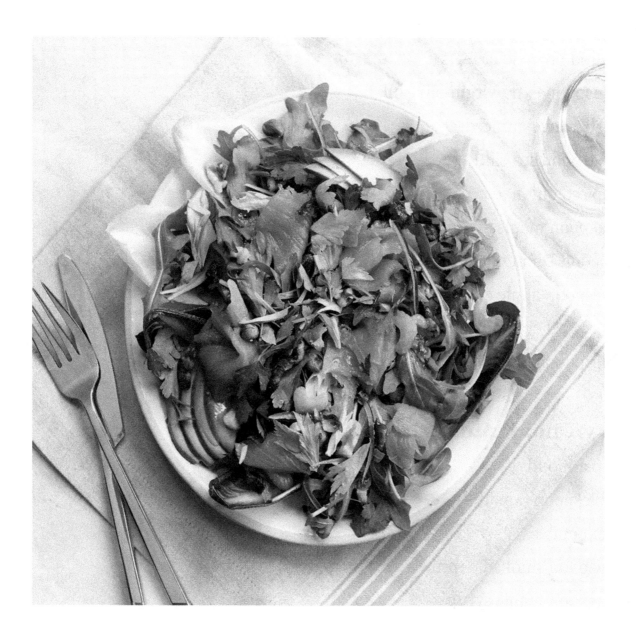

Broccoli Salad

This Broccoli Salad is the perfect easy cookout side dish! Tangy, refreshing and full of sweet/salty flavor!

Ingredients: 2 servings

- ½ pound broccoli crowns
- 1 tablespoon extra virgin olive oil
- ½ garlic clove, minced
- 1/8 teaspoon sea salt
- ¼ cup red onion, diced
- ½ teaspoon maple syrup
- 1 teaspoon Dijon mustard
- 1 tablespoon apple cider vinegar
- ¼ cup dried cranberries
- 1 tablespoon mayo

Smoky Tamari Almond:

- ¼ cup almond
- ½ tablespoon tamari
- ¼ cup pepitas
- ¼ teaspoon smoked paprika
- ¼ teaspoon maple syrup

Directions:

- Preheat the oven to 350° F and line a baking sheet with parchment paper.

- Chop the broccoli florets into ½ inch pieces and any remaining stems into ¼ inch dice. Peel any woody or course parts from the stem first.

- In the bottom of a large bowl, whish together the olive oil, mayo, mustard, apple cider vinegar, maple syrup, garlic, and salt. Add the broccoli, onions, and cranberries and toss to coat.

- Place the almonds and pepitas on the baking sheet, toss with the tamari, maple syrup, and smoked paprika and spread into a thin layer. Bake 10 to 14 minutes or until golden brown. Remove from the oven and let cool for 5 minutes.

- Toss the almonds and pepitas into the salad, reserving a few to sprinkle on top.

Nutritional info per serving: Calories 212, Fat 15g, Carbohydrates 32g, Protein 9g

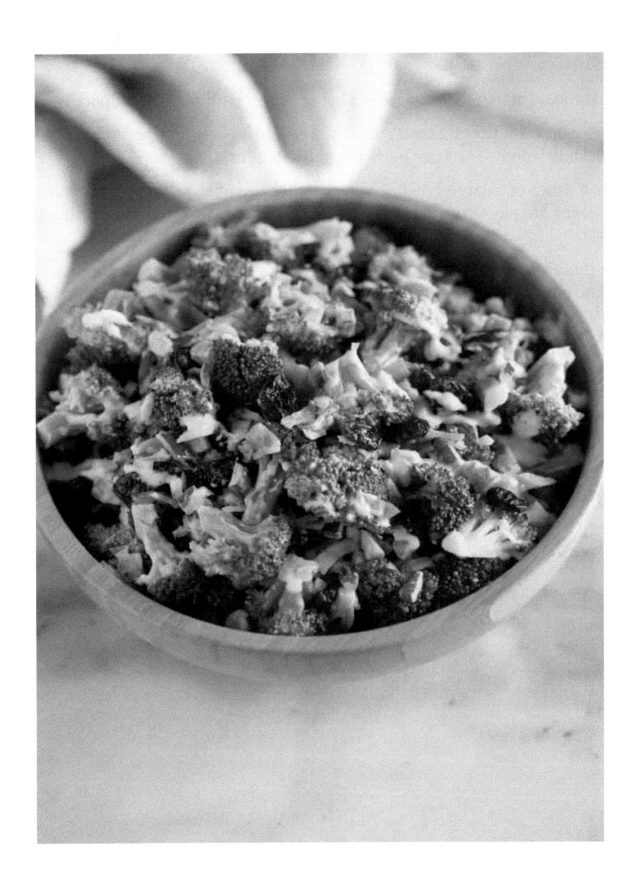

Buckwheat Stir Fry with Kale, Peppers & Artichokes

Buckwheat Stir Fry recipe with cooked roasted buckwheat groats, kale, pepper, marinated artichoke sand optional feta cheese for a healthy meal!

Ingredients: 4 servings

Buckwheat:

- 1 cup roasted roasted buckwheat groats, uncooked
- 2 cups water
- Pinch of salt

Stir Fry:

- ½ bunch kale, ribs removed and finely chopped
- 2 large bell peppers, cut into strips
- 1 cup marinated artichoke hearts, drained and chopped
- 2 large garlic cloves, minced
- ¼ cup parsley, finely chopped
- ¼ cup basil, finely chopped
- 2 tablespoons coconut oil
- 1 teaspoon salt

Directions:

Buckwheat:

- In a medium pot, add buckwheat. Rinse and drain with cold water a few times. Add 2 cups water and a pinch of salt. Cover and bring to a boil. Reduce heat to low and cook for 15 minutes. Do not open the lid. Remove from heat, let stand for 3 minutes abd fluff with a fork.

Stir Fry:

• In the meanwhile, preheat a non-stick wok on medium heat and swirl ½ tablespoon of oil to coat. Add garlic and sautè for 10 seconds. Add kale and 1/8 teaspoon salt. Sautè until shrunk in half, stirring occasionally. Transfer to a medium bowl.

• Return wok to high heat and swirl ½ tablespoon of oil. Add peppers and 1/8 teaspoon salt. Sautè until golden brown, stirring occasionally. Transfer to a bowl with kale.

• Reduce heat to low and add remaining 1 tablespoon of oil. Add cooked buckwheat and briefly stir it to coat in oil. Turn off heat. Add previously cooked kale and peppers, artichoke hearts, basil, parsley, and remaining ¼ teaspoon salt. Stir gently and serve warm!

Nutritional info per serving: Calories 258, Fat 11.9g, Carbohydrates 35.2g, Protein 6.8g

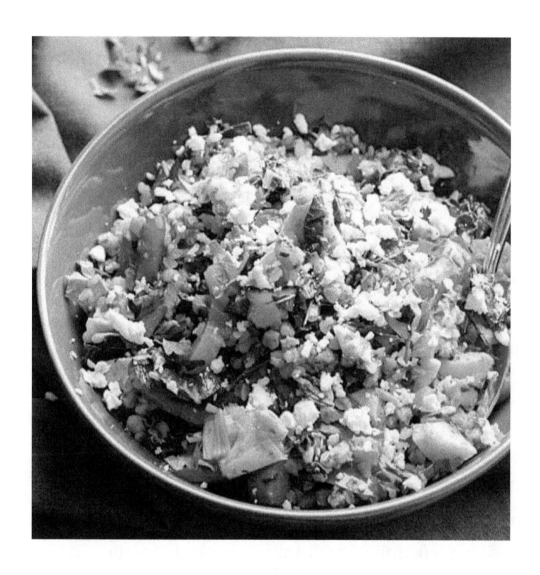

Arugula, Egg, and Charred Asparagus Salad

Just a hint of char on the asparagus adds fantastic complexity to this simple 5-ingredient spring salad!

Ingredients: 4 servings

- 12 oz medium asparagus, trimmed
- ½ teaspoon black pepper, divided
- 4 large eggs in shells
- 1 tablespoon fresh lemon juice
- 5 oz baby arugula
- 1 tablespoon extra virgin olive oil
- 1 tablespoon water
- ¼ cup plain whole-milk Greek yogurt
- 1 teaspoon kosher salt, divided

Directions:

- Preheat broiler to high.

- Bring a small saucepan filled with water to a boil. Carefully add eggs. Cook 8 minutes. Place eggs in a bowl filled with ice water and let stand for 2 minutes. Peel eggs, cut into quarters, and sprinkle with ¼ teaspoon salt and 1/8 teaspoon pepper.

- Combine olive oil, ¼ teaspoon salt, ¼ teaspoon pepper, and asparagus on a baking sheet. Spread in a single layer in pan. Broil 3 minutes or until lightly charred. Remove asparagus mixture from pan and cut into 2 inch pieces.

- Combine remaining ¼ teaspoon salt, remaining 1/8 teaspoon pepper, yogurt, juice, and 1 tablespoon water in a medium bowl, stirring with a whisk. Add arugula and toss. Arrange arugula mixture on a platter. Top with asparagus mixture and eggs. Enjoy!

Nutritional info per serving: Calories 147, Fat 9.1g, Carbohydrates 6g, Protein 10g

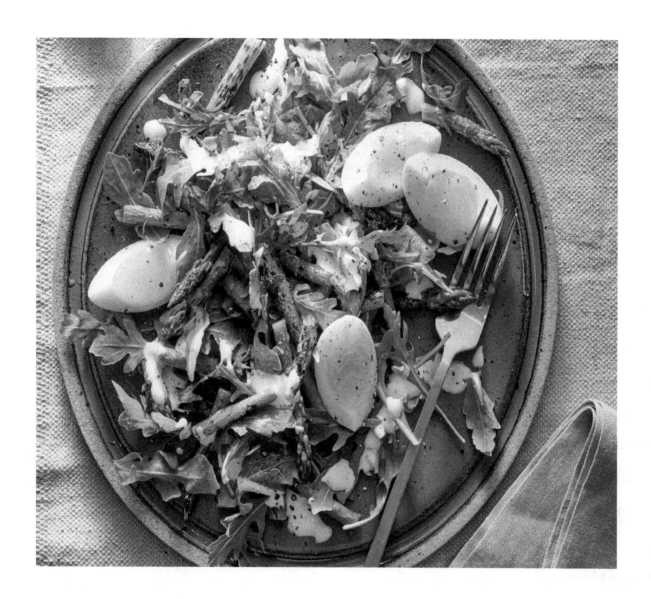

Spring Vegetable and Quinoa Salad with Bacon

This rich and dynamic quinoa salad could easily be pulled together with whatever leftover grain you have on hand, such as farro or bulgur!

Ingredients: 4 servings

- 1 ¾ cups ginger-coconut quinoa
- 2,5 cups fresh asparagus, cut diagonally into 1 inch pieces
- 3 center-cut bacon slices, chopped
- 1 tablespoon unsalted butter
- 3 tablespoons cider vinegar
- ½ cup frozen green peas
- 2 teaspoons whole-grain Dijon mustard
- 5 oz baby spinach
- 3 tablespoons sliced almonds, toasted
- 1 teaspoon black pepper
- 1 tablespoon fresh thyme leaves
- 1 tablespoon chopped fresh tarragon
- ½ cup chopped fresh flat-leaf parsley

Directions:

- Bring a large saucepan filled with water to a boil. Add asparagus and peas. Boil 2 minutes, then drain. Plunge into a bowl of ice water. Drain.
- Cook bacon in a large skillet over medium-high heat 4 minutes, stirring occasionally. Remove bacon from pan with a slotted spoon. Set aside. Add vinegar, butter, and Dijon mustard to drippings in pan, stirring with a whisk until butter melts. Add quinoa and pepper to pan. Cook 1 minute. Place quinoa mixture in a medium

bowl. Add asparagus mixture, parsley, tarragon, thyme, and spinach, tossing to combine. Divide quinoa mixture among 4 plates; sprinkle evenly with reserved bacon and almonds.

Nutritional info per serving: Calories 263, Fat 9.8g, Carbohydrates 28g, Protein 7g

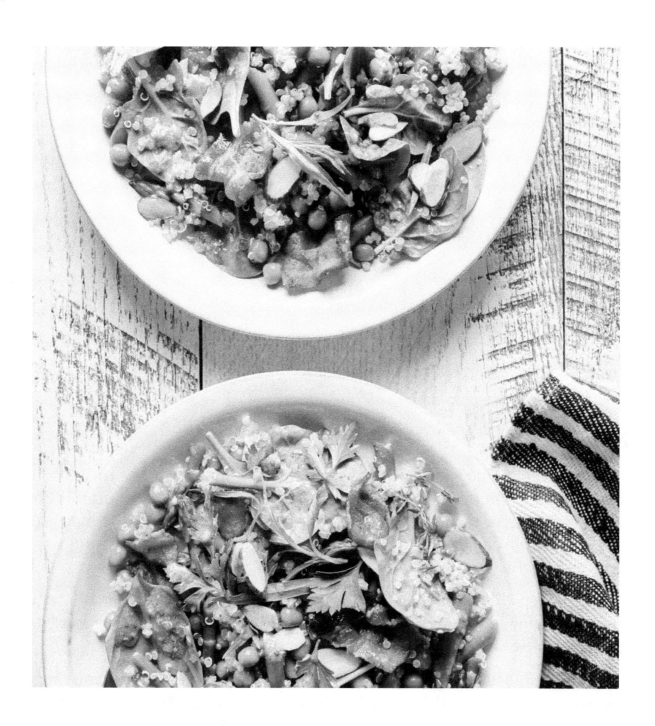

Golden Chicory in Prosciutto Wraps

Try this simplified version of the traditional French one! You could use normal sliced honey roast ham if you prefer!

Ingredients: 1 serving

- 2 head of chicory
- 4 slices prosciutto or Serrano ham
- 75 ml vegetable stock, or white wine
- 2 tablespoons butter
- 2 tablespoons Dijon mustard
- ¼ cup whipping cream
- 2 thyme sprigs
- 4 slices, about 2 oz melting cheese (cheddar is great)
- Sautèed potatoes and green salad, to serve

Directions:

- Preheat the oven to 350° F. Cut a cross from the base halfway to the tip of each head of chicory. Stuff the butter into the slits, then lay the slices of prosciutto or Serrano ham in pairs on the work surface, overlapping them slightly. Paint the ham with the mustard and lay the chicory on top. Roll each chicory head away from you, wrapping it snugly in the ham.

- Lay the wrapped chicory in a small ovenproof dish or pan, pour over the vegetable stock or white wine on top with the thyme sprigs. Cover the dish with a loose tent of foil and bake for 30-40 minutes until the chicory is softened.

- Uncover the dish, lay the cheese slices over the chicory and bake, still uncovered, for a further 6-8 minutes, until the cheese is melting and golden. The chicory is now ready to serve. For an extra touch, remove the chicory, place the pan on a medium heat and boil the juices with the cream for 4-5 minutes until rich and syrupy. Pour the sauce over the chicory. Serve with sautèed potatoes and salad.

Nutritional info per serving: Calories 493, Fat 36g, Carbohydrates 9g, Protein 32g

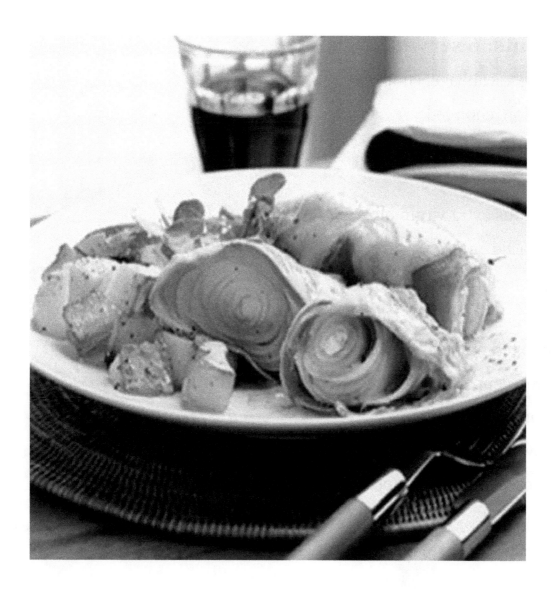

Vegetable Cabbage Soup

This is one of the most adaptable soup! It's flavorful, super healthy, and comes together in no time!

Ingredients: 6 servings

- ½ large head cabbage, chopped
- 1 large onion, chopped
- 2 stalks celery, minced
- 2 carrots, chopped
- 2 tablespoons extra virgin olive oil
- 2 cloves garlic, minced
- ½ teaspoon chili powder
- 1 can white beans, drained and rinsed
- 1 can chopped fire-roasted tomatoes
- 1 pinch red pepper flakes
- 1 teaspoon thyme leaves
- 4 cups low-sodium vegetable broth
- 2 tablespoons freshly chopped parsley, plus more for garnish
- Kosher salt
- Freshly ground black pepper
- 2 cups water

Directions:

- In a large pot over medium heat, heat olive oil. Add onion, celery, and carrots, and season with salt, pepper, and chili powder. Cook, stirring often, until vegetables are soft, 5 to 6 minutes. Stir in beans, thyme, and garlic and cook until garlic is fragrant, about 30 seconds. Add broth and water, and bring to a simmer.

• Stir in tomatoes and cabbage and simmer until cabbage is wilted, about 6 minutes.

• Remove from heat and stir in red pepper flakes, and parsley. Season to taste with salt and pepper. Garnish with more parsley, if desired. Enjoy!

Nutritional info per serving: Calories 92, Fat 0.8g, Carbohydrates 11.6, Protein 2.5g

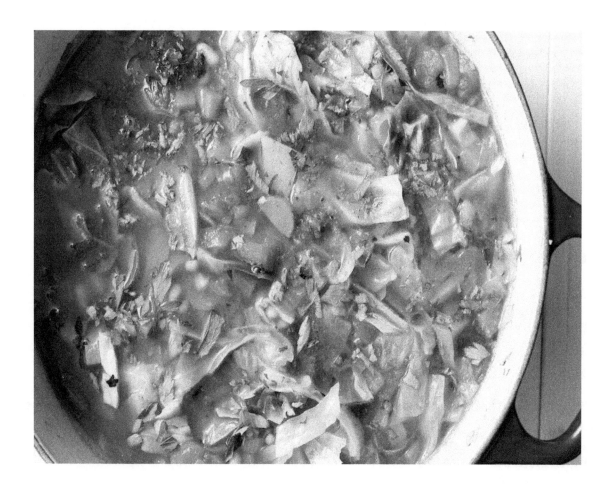

Fresh Herb Frittata

Frittatas are literally one of the easiest recipes to make! Enjoy this tasty Fresh Herb Frittata!

Ingredients: 6 servings

- 8 fresh eggs
- 3 tablespoons chopped fresh parsley
- 2 tablespoons chopped fresh oregano
- 4 scallions, slice thin, using both white and green parts
- ½ cup heavy cream
- ¾ cup finely grated parmesan cheese, divided into ½ cup and 1/4 cup portions
- Salt and pepper to taste

Directions:

- Preheat oven to 400° F.
- In a medium mixing bowl combine eggs, parsley, scallions, oregano, ½ cup of cheese, and heavy cream. Whisk together until thoroughly combined. Season with salt and pepper, to taste.
- In a well-seasoned 10 inch cast iron skillet, heat about 1 tablespoon of olive oil over medium heat.
- Add egg mixture and cook for about 5 minutes, or until edges start to set.
- Sprinkle remaining ¼ cup of cheese on the top of the eggs.
- Transfer skillet to the oven and bake for 10-12 minutes, or until frittata is piffed up, edges are browned, and it jiggles just slightly in the center.
- Broil on low for about 30-45 seconds to further brown the cheese topping.

Nutritional info per serving: Calories 105, Fat 2.8g, Carbohydrates 5g, Protein 7g

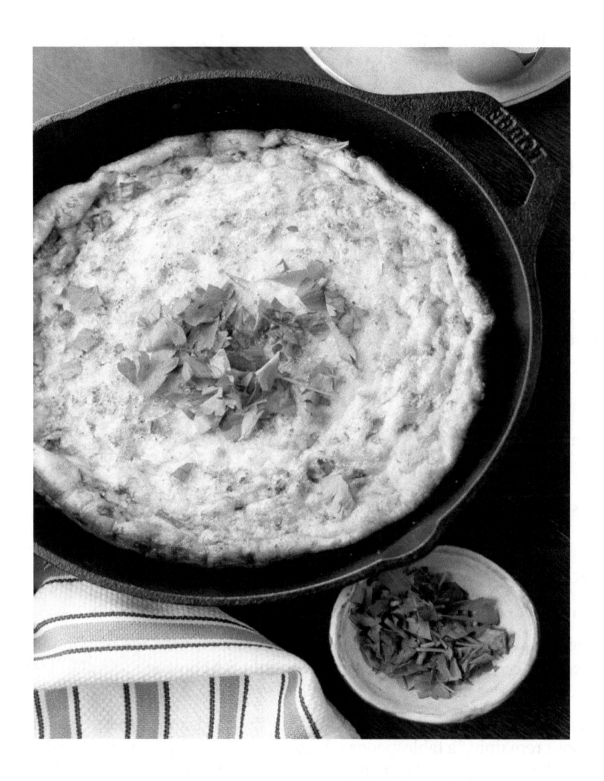

Grilled Aparagus with Caper Vinaigrette

Grilling adds flavor to the asparagus, as does the tangy caper vinaigrette that's drizzled over the spears!

Ingredients: 6 servings

- 1 ½ pounds asparagus spears, trimmed
- 2 teaspoons caper, coarsely chopped
- 1 tablespoon red wine vinegar
- 1 garlic clove, minced
- 3 tablespoons extra virgin olive oil
- ¼ cup small basil leaves
- ½ teaspoon Dijon mustard
- Cooking spray
- ½ teaspoon kosher salt, divided
- ¼ teaspoon freshly ground black pepper

Directions:

- Preheat grill to medium-high heat.

- Place asparagus in a shallow dish. Add 1 tablespoon oil and ¼ teaspoon salt, tossing well to coat. Place asparagus on grill rack coated with cooking spray. Grill 4 minutes or until crisp-tender, turning after 2 minutes.

- Combine remaining ¼ teaspoon salt, vinegar, mustard, and garlic. Stir with a whisk. Slowly pour remaining 2 tablespoons oil into vinegar mixture, stirring constantly with a whisk. Stir in capers. Arrange asparagus on a serving platter. Drizzle with vinaigrette, and sprinkle with basil.

Nutritional info per serving: Calories 89, Fat 6.9g, Carbohydrates 4.7g, Protein 2.8g

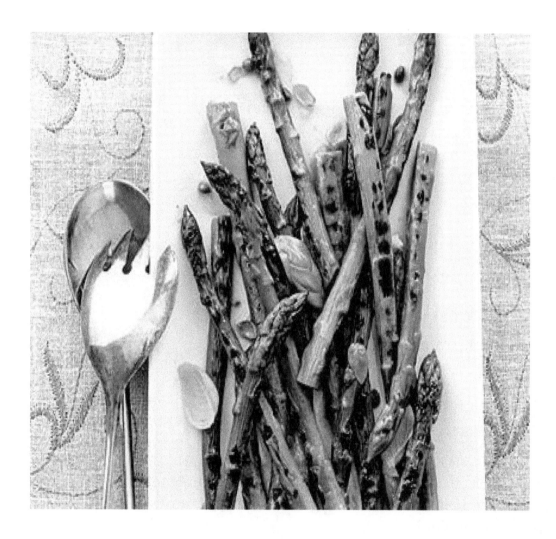

Herby Pork with Apple & Chicory Salad

A healthy crisp salad with a low-fat cut of herb-crusted pork!

Ingredients: 4 servings

- 14 oz pork tenderloin, trimmed of any fat and sinew
- 2 large apples, cored and sliced
- 270g pack chicory, leaves separated
- 1 tablespoon honey
- 1 tablespoon walnut oil
- 1 tablespoon chopped parsley
- 1 tablespoon chopped tarragon
- 2 teaspoons wholegrain mustard
- Juice of 1 lemon

Directions:

- Heat oven to 350° F. Rub the pork with 1 teaspoon oil, 1 teaspoon mustard and some seasoning. Brown, transfer to a baking tray and press on half the herbs. Roast for 15 minutes until just cooked.

- To make the salad, mix the lemon juice, honey and remaining walnut oil and mustard together. Season and toss through the apples, chicory and remaining herbs. Serve the pork sliced, with the salad on the side.

Nutritional info per serving: Calories 252, Fat 8g, Carbohydrates 16g, Protein 22g

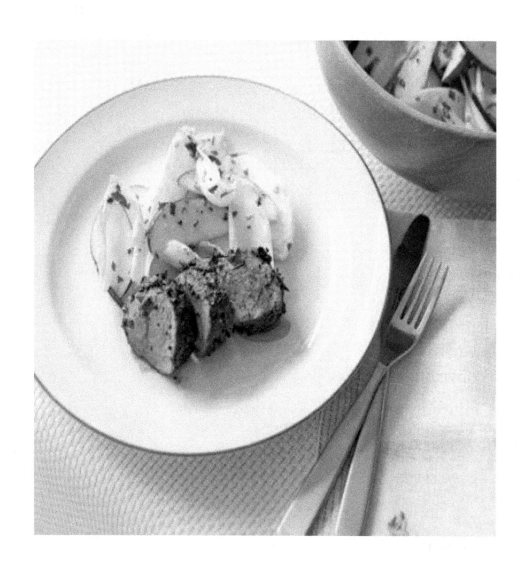

Chia, Quinoa & Avocado Salad

A super salad that's ready in just 30 minutes! This protein-rich mix of quinoa, feta, sunflower and chia seeds is all dressed up with lime and chilies and comes topped with creamy chunks of avocado.

Ingredients: 2 servings

- ½ cup quinoa
- ¼ cup black chia seeds
- 1 avocado
- ¾ cup feta cheese
- 1 red onion
- 1 chili
- 2 tablespoons olive oil
- 1 garlic clove, minced
- 1/8 cup sunflower seeds
- 1 tablespoon agave syrup
- 2 limes
- ½ cup cherry tomatoes
- 1 cup rocket
- Sea salt
- Freshly ground pepper

Directions:

- Tip the quinoa into a sieve and rinse under cold water for a few minutes to rinse off the soapy coating. Tip into a pan. Pur in 1 cup boiling water. Cover and bring to a boil.

Turn the heat right down and simmer for 10-12 minutes until the water has been absorbed and the quinoa is tender. Take off the heat.

• While the quinoa simmers, tip the chia seeds into a dry frying pan. Toast over a medium heat for 3-4 minutes until the chia seeds smell aromatic. Tip into a large bowl. Add the sunflower seeds to the frying pan and toast fro 2 minutes. Add the chia seeds intp the bowl. Stir the quinoa into the bowl.

• Peel and dice the red onion. Quarter the cherry tomatoes. Add them to the bowl. Halve the avocado. Scoop out the stone, then scoop the flesh from the skin. Roughly chop it and add to the bowl. Roughly chop the rocket leaves and add them to the bowl too. Toss everything together.

• Juice the limes into a small bowl. Add the olive oil and agave syrup. Halve the chili. Flick out the seeds and white bits for less heat and finely chop the chilies. Peel and crush the garlic. Add to the lime juice with a pinch of salt and pepper. Whisk to make a dressing.

• Add the dressing to the bowl. Toss to mix. Heap the salad up on serving plates and crumble over the feta to serve.

Nutritional info per serving: Calories 212, Fat 11g, Carbohydrates 29g, Protein 8g

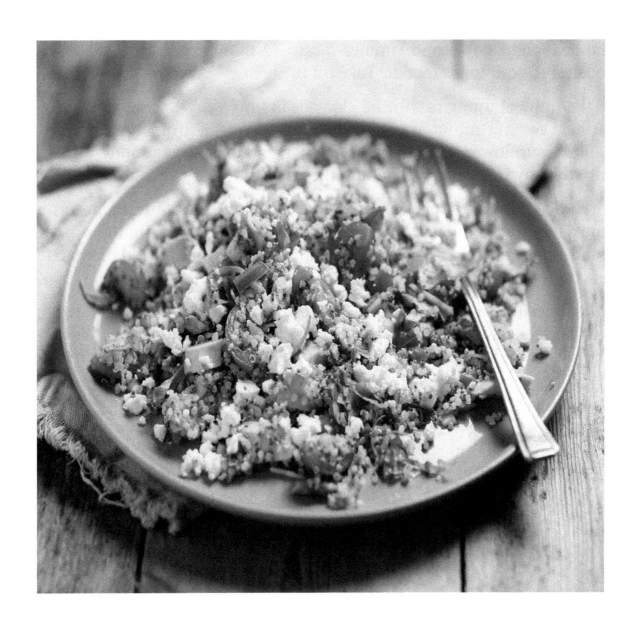

Tomato Green Bean Soup

This colorful soup is delicious any time of the year!

Ingredients: 4 servings

- 1 ½ cups diced fresh tomatoes
- ½ cup chopped onion
- ½ pound fresh green beans, cut into 1 inch pieces
- ½ cup chopped carrots
- 1/8 cup minced fresh basil
- ½ garlic clove, minced
- ¼ teaspoon salt
- 1/8 teaspoon pepper
- 1 teaspoon butter
- 3 cups reduced-sodium vegetable broth

Directions:

- In a large saucepan, sautè onion and carrots in butter for 5 minutes. Stir in the broth, green beans and garlic. Bring to a boil. Reduce heat. Cover and simmer for 20 minutes or until vegetables are tender.
- Stir in the tomatoes, basil, salt and pepper. Cover and simmer 5 minutes longer.

Nutritional info per serving: Calories 57, Fat 1.3g, Carbohydates 10g, Protein 5g

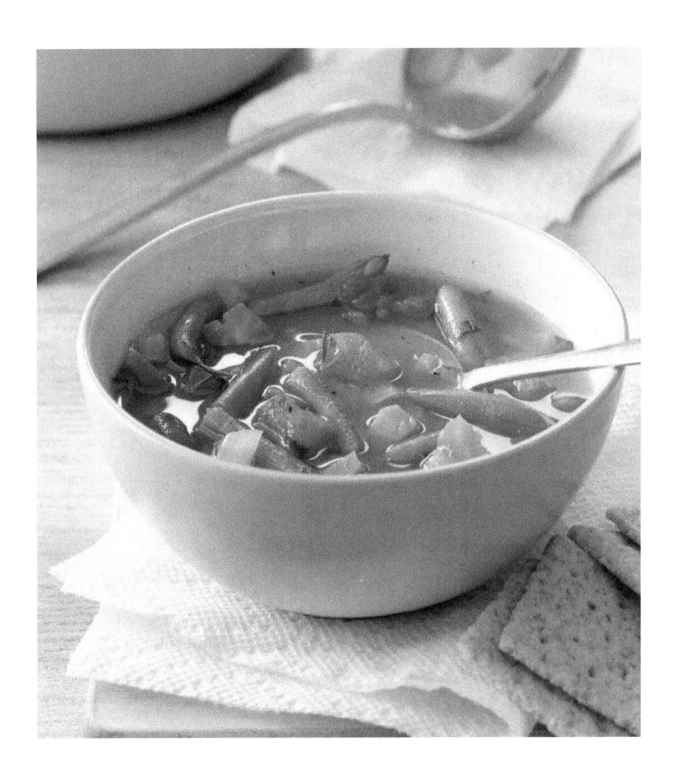

Kale Salad with Pecorino and Lemon

This salad is so simple: just kale, Pecorino Romano, and a light vinaigrette!

Ingredients: 4 servings

- 1 large bunch kale, washed and trimmed of steams
- 2 lemons, juiced
- 4 oz Pecorino Romano, grated
- ½ cup olive oil
- Kosher salt and fresh black pepper to taste

Directions:

- Roll several kale leaves lengthwise and using the point of a knife, cut away the thick center steam. Discard. Roll the remaining stack of de-veined leaves into a tight cigar shape and slice into thin ribbons.

- Toss the shaved kale with the cheese. Whisk the lemon juice and olive oil and pour over the salad. Taste and season with salt and pepper. Let the salad sit at room temperature for an hour before serving.

Nutritional info per serving: Calories 238, Fat 15g, Carbohydrates 21g, Protein 8g

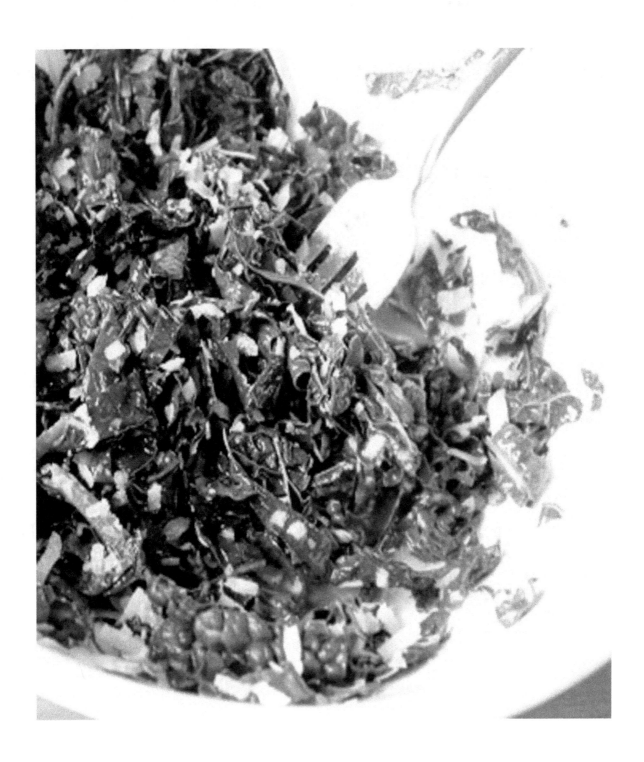

Tahini-Date Salted Caramels

These Tahini-Date Salted Caramels have a great creamy and chewy texture! They also come together really easily and don't require any time on the stovetop!

Ingredients: 18 candies

- 1 cup pitted dates
- ½ cup tahini
- ½ teaspoon ground cardamom
- 2 tablespoons coconut oil
- 1/8 teaspoon salt

Directions:

- Combine the dates, tahini, coconut oil, and cardamom in a blender or food processor. You should have a very smooth, creamy, and thick paste.

- Transfer the mixture to a parchment-lined loaf pan and use a spatula to press it down evenly. Sprinkle with salt.

- Freeze until firm. Remove from the pan and cut into bite-size pieces.

Nutritional info per serving: Calories 132, Fat 7.5g, Carbohydrates 22.5g, Protein 4.1g

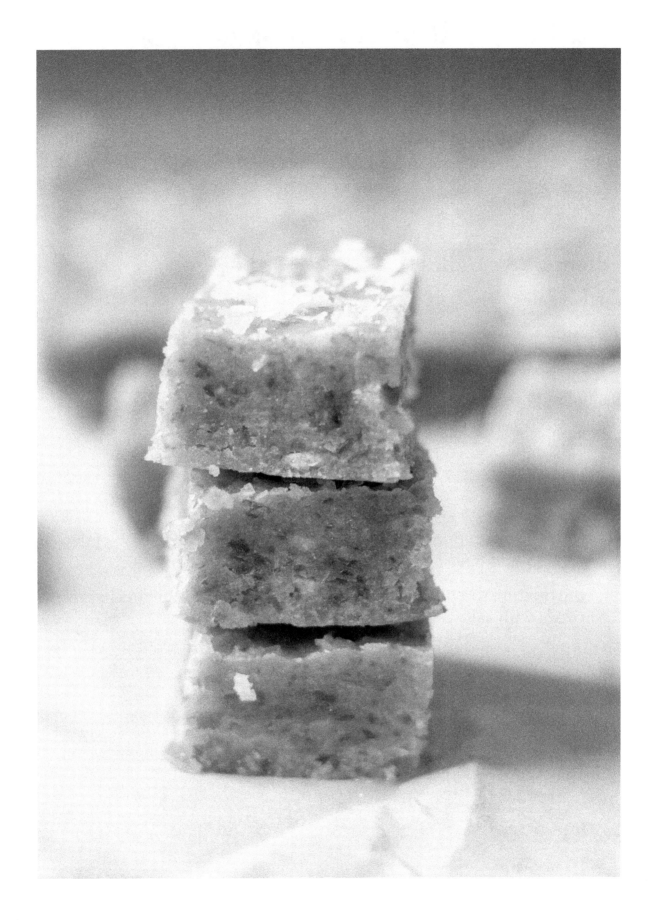

Bacon-Wrapped Dates

If you've never wrapped a date in bacon, you don't know what you're missing!

Ingredients: 20 to 24 bites

- 12 to 16 oz bacon
- 20 to 24 toasted almonds
- 20 to 24 Medjool dates
- 4 oz goat cheese or blue cheese

Directions:

- Arrange a rack in the middle of the oven and heat to 400° F. Line a baking sheet with parchment or a silicone baking mat and set aside.

- Use a paring knife to cut a slit in the side of each date. Use your thumbs to open the date slightly. Remove the pits if your dates still have them inside.

- Use a spoon to stuff a little goat cheese or blue cheese into each date. Use the back of the spoon to press the cheese into the date. If you're adding almonds, press an almond or two into the cheese. Press the date closed.

- Cut the strips of bacon in half crosswise. Wrap each date with a half-strip of bacon. Secure the end of the bacon with a toothpick.

- Place the stuffed date on its side on the baking sheet. Repeat with the remaining dates, spacing them evenly apart. Bake the dates for 15 minutes.

- Flip the dates. Keep an eye on the dates and remove from the oven as soon as the bacon is as crispy as you like it, 15 to 20 minutes more.

- If the dates seem greasy, blot the sides as well as the bottoms with paper towels. Serve warm or room temperature. Enjoy!

Nutritional info per serving: Calories 226, Fat 13.2g, Carbohydrates 19.9g, Protein 6.8

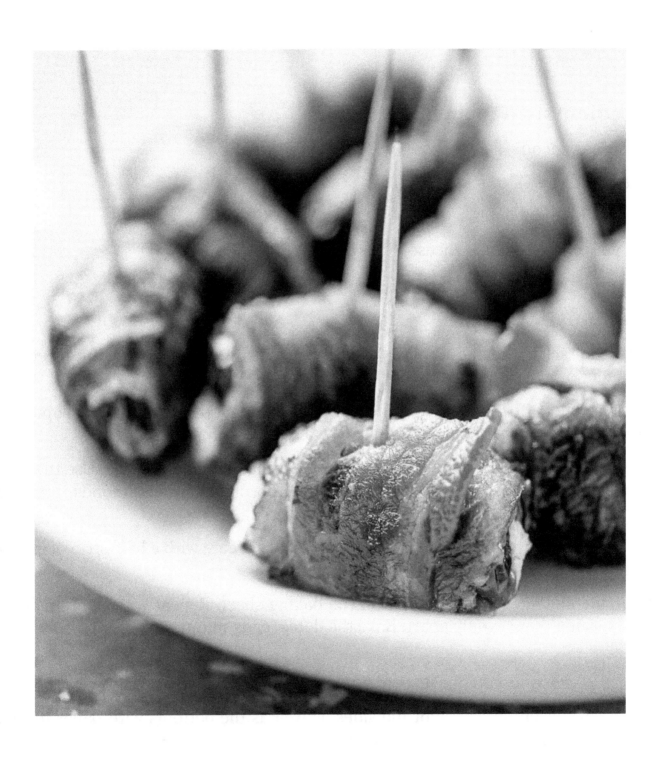

Avocado Tuna Salad

This Avocado Tuna Salad is so simple and flavorful! Definitely an upgrade on classic tuna salad!

Ingredients: 6 servings

- 15 oz tuna in oil, drained and flaked
- 3 medium avocados, peeled, pitted and sliced
- 1 cucumber, sliced
- ¼ cup cilantro
- 1 red onion, thinly sliced
- 2 tablespoons extra virgin olive oil
- 2 tablespoons lemon juice, freshly squeezed
- 1 teaspoon sea salt
- 1/8 teaspoon black pepper

Directions:

- In a large bowl, combine cucumber, avocado, red onion, tuna, and ¼ cup cilantro.
- Drizzle salad ingredients with 2 tablespoons lemon juice, 2 tablespoons olive oil, 1 teaspoon salt, and 1/8 teaspoon black pepper. Toss to combine and serve. Enjoy!

Nutritional info per serving: Calories 289, Fat 18g, Carbohydrates 8.7g, Protein 22g

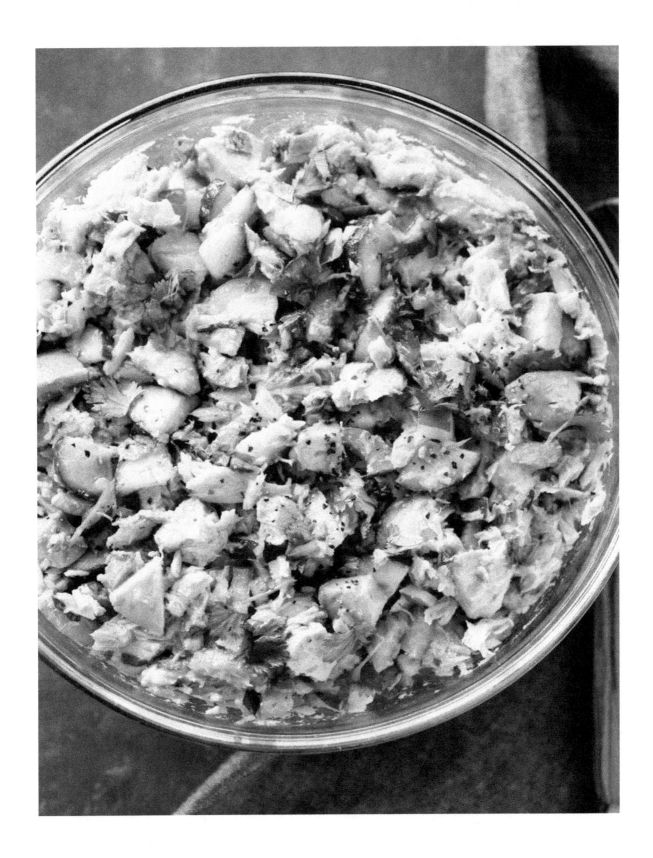

Herb-Roasted Olives and Tomatoes

Eat these roasted veggies with a crunchy baguette or a couple of cheeses!

Ingredients: 4 cups

- 1 cup Greek olives
- 1 cup garlic-stuffed olives
- 2 cups cherry tomatoes
- 1 cup pitted ripe olives
- 1 tablespoon herbs de Provence
- 3 tablespoons olive oil
- 8 garlic cloves, peeled
- ¼ teaspoon pepper

Directions:

- Preheat oven to 425° F.

- Combine cherry tomatoes, garlic-stuffed olives, Greek olives, pitted ripe olives, and garlic cloves on a greased baking pan. Add oil and seasonings. Toss to coat. Roast until tomatoes are softened, 15-20 minutes, stirring occasionally.

Nutritional info per serving (1/4 cup): Calories 69, Fat 6g, Carbohydrates 3g, Protein 0.5g

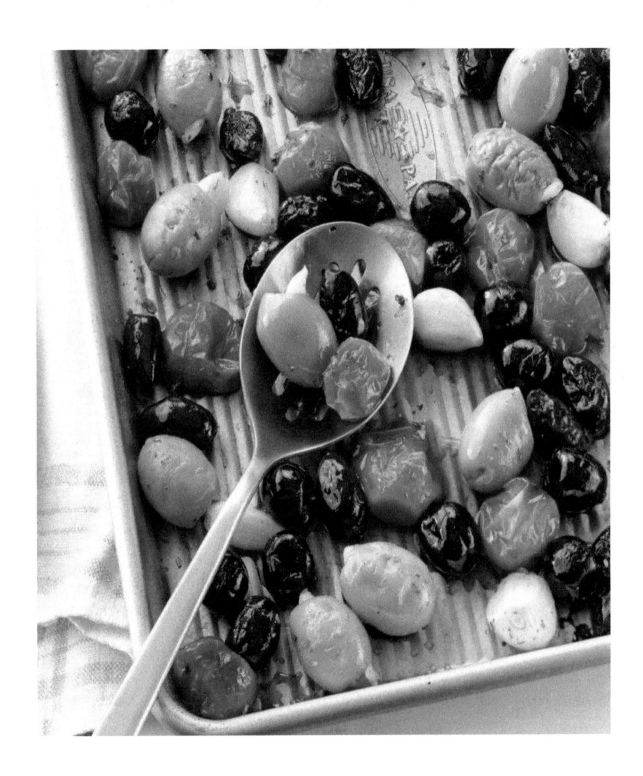

Roasted Red Onions Stuffed with Mascarpone Cheese

Mascarpone is an Italian cheese with a delicate, fresh smell that lightens up all dishes! And this recipe is so sweet and simple you wonder why you haven't had it before!

Ingredients: 4 servings

- 4 large red onions
- 1 cup mascarpone cheese
- 1 shallot, diced
- 4 cloves garlic, minced
- 1 teaspoon minced fresh thyme

Directions:

- Preheat oven to 425° F.
- Cut both ends off onions and place onto a baking sheet. Roast in preheated oven until centers are soft, about 15 minutes. Remove, and let onions cool.
- Reduce heat to 350° F.
- Peel onions and remove center core leaving ½ inch outer shell intact. Mince the center flesh and place in a bowl. Combine with mascarpone cheese, shallot, garlic, and thyme. Fill onion shells with cheese mixture and replace onto baking sheet.
- Bake until the surface of the cheese bubbles, about 10 minutes. Serve hot!

Nutritional info per serving: Calories 302, Fat 23.2g, Carbohydrates 16.3g, Protein 5.9g

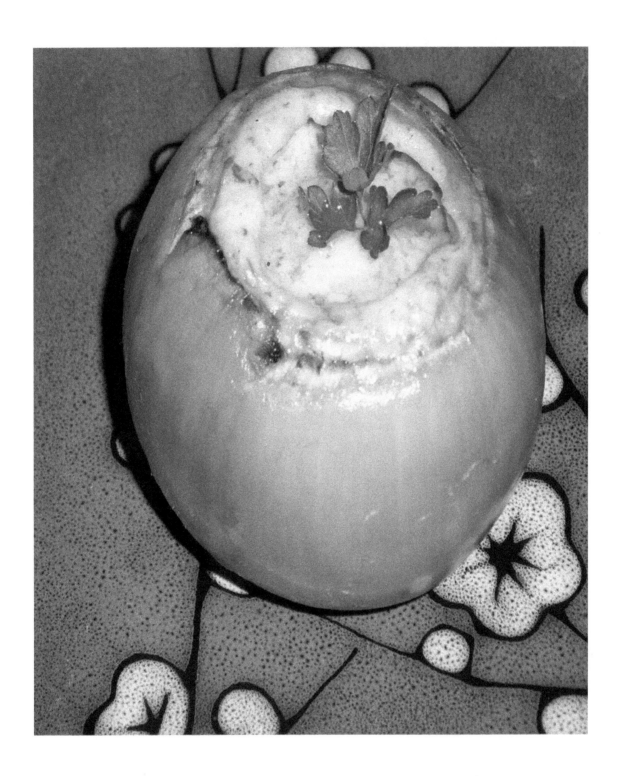

Mixed Olive Crostini

These little toasts are pretty and irresistible! They're always a big hit!

Ingredients: 2 dozen

- 1 can chopped ripe olives
- ½ cup Parmesan cheese, grated
- 1 French bread baguette
- ½ cup pimento-stuffed olives, finely chopped
- 1 tablespoon olive oil
- 2 garlic cloves, minced
- ¼ cup butter, softened
- ¾ cup shredded part-skim mozzarella cheese
- ¼ cup minced fresh parsley

Directions:

- In a small bowl, combine chopped ripe olives, pimento-stuffed olives, grated Parmesan cheese, butter, olive oil, and garlic cloves. Stir in mozzarella cheese and parsley. Cut baguette into 24 slices. Place on an ungreased baking sheet. Spread with olive mixture.
- Broil for 2-3 minutes or until edges are lightly browned and cheese is melted.

Nutritional info per serving: Calories 102, Fat 5.8g, Carbohydrates 10.2g, Protein 3g

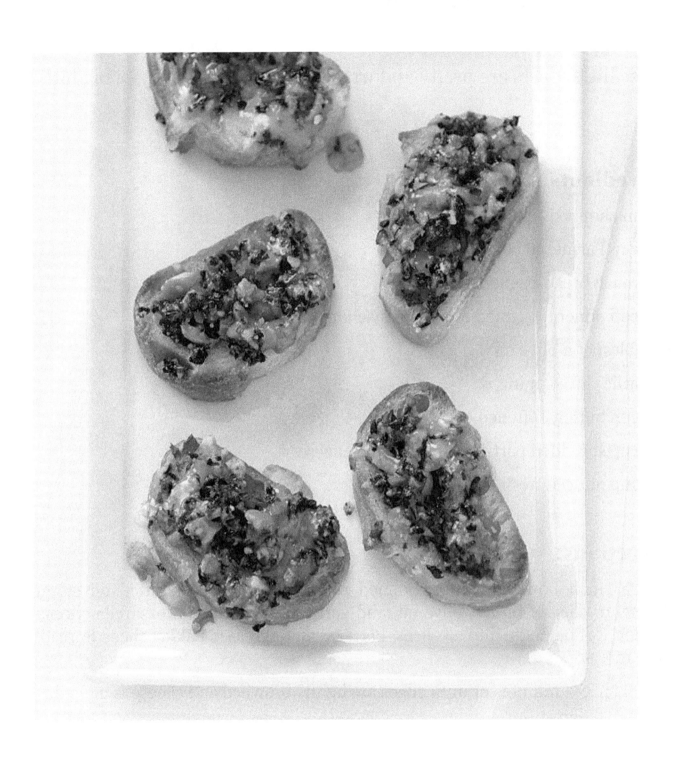

Cannellini Bean Soup

Cannellini beans bring tremendous flavour to this soup!

Ingredients: 4 servings

- 1 ½ cups dry cannellini beans
- 1 onion, chopped
- 3 small long carrots, peeled, halved lengthwise, and sliced
- 2 cloves garlic, minced
- 2 tablespoons extra virgin olive oil, plus more for drizzling
- 1/8 cup fresh basil leaves
- ¼ cup chopped tomatoes
- 1/8 cup chopped fresh flat-leaf parsley
- 2 celery stalks, peeled and chopped
- Freshly grated Parmesan cheese
- 1 tablespoon coarse salt
- Freshly ground black pepper

Directions:

- Rinse the beans well and place in a large pot. Cover the beans with 4 quarts of water. Bring to a boil, cover, and turn off the heat. Allow to soak for 1 hour.

- Place the olive oil, onions, and garlic in a large heavy-bottomed pot over medium heat. When the garlic begins to sizzle, after about 30 seconds, add the carrots and celery and continue to cook, stirring, for about 5 minutes. Stir in the tomatoes, basil, and parsley and cook, stirring occasionally, for an additional 3 minutes.

- Add the soaked beans, cover with cold water, and stir to combine. Bring to a boil, reduce the heat, and simmer, partially covered, until the beans are tender and creamy, at least 1 ½ hours up to 2,5 hours. Add water if necessary to achieve desired consistency; the soup should be thick. Add the salt halfway through the cooking. Serve with freshly grated Parmesan cheese, freshly ground black pepper, and a drizzle of olive oil.

Nutritional info per serving: Calories 314, Fat 9g, Carbohydrates 46g, Protein 22g

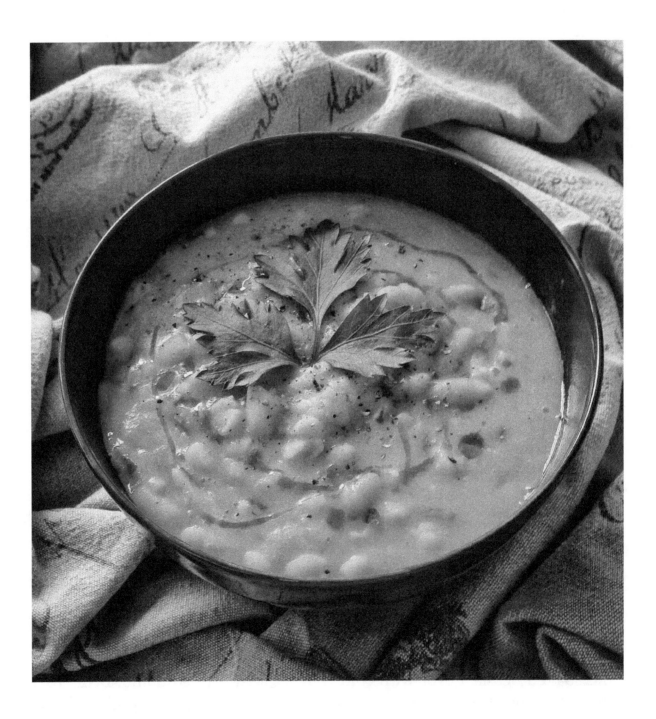

Celery Caesar Salad

Taste this great fresh and flavourful version of the Caesar Salad!

Ingredients: 4 servings

- 1 medium celery root, peeled
- 4 celery stalks, sliced in half lengthwise, thinly cut on a diagonal, plus about ½ cup celery leaves
- 3 oil-packed anchovy fillets, divided
- 2 slices 2 inch thick country-style bread, crusts removed, torn into bite-size pieces
- 1 large egg yolk
- ½ lemon
- 2 tablespoons fresh lemon juice
- 1 garlic clove, peeled
- 8 tablespoons olive oil, divided
- 2 oz Parmesan cheese, shaved
- Kosher salt
- Freshly ground black pepper

Directions:

- Preheat oven to 400° F. Toss bread with 2 tablespoons oil on a rimmed baking sheet. Season with salt. Bake, tossing halfway through, until golden brown and crisp, about 8-10 minutes. Set croutons aside.

- Thinly slice celery root into thin matchsticks. Place in a large bowl and add enough water to cover. Squeeze in juice from lemon.

• Purèe egg yolk, lemon juice, garlic, and 1 anchovy fillet in a blender until smooth. With motor running, gradually drizzle in 3 tablespoons oil, then 1 ½ tablespoons water, followed by remaining 3 tablespoons oil. Season dressing with salt and pepper.

• Drain reserved celery root and toss with celery in a large bowl. Chop remaining 2 anchovy fillets and add to bowl along with celery leaves, Parmesan cheese, croutons, and dressing and toss to combine. Enjoy!

Nutritional info per serving: Calories 352, Fat 28g, Carbohydrates 14g, Protein 7g

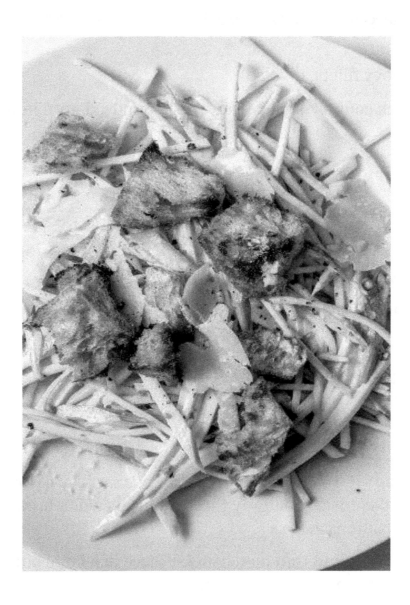

Orange, Almond & Date Salad

I love the combination of oranges and dates! Enjoy this amazing salad!

Ingredients: 4 servings

- ¼ cup raw almonds
- 4 dates, thinly sliced
- 4 to 6 oranges, depending on size
- 1 teaspoon coconut oil, melted
- 1 teaspoon agave nectar
- ¼ teaspoon orange flower water
- ¼ teaspoon cinnamon
- 1 tablespoon chiffonade of mint
- Salt

Directions:

- Preheat oven to 325° F. In a small bowl, combine coconut oil, agave nectar, cinnamon, and a smidgen of salt. Add almonds and toss to coat. Spread almonds in a single layer on a parchment-lined baking sheet. Bake, stirring once or twice, until toasted, about 10 minutes. Cool before using.

- Slice the ends off each orange. Stand each orange upright and cut away the peel and pith, following the curve of the orange. Cut each orange into ¼ inch thick rounds and remove any seeds.

- Arrange the orange slices on a platter. Drizzle with orange flower water, if using. Scatter dates, almonds, and mint on top, and serve!

Nutritional info per serving: Calories 201, Fat 5.8g, Carbohydrates 36.7g, Protein 4.1g

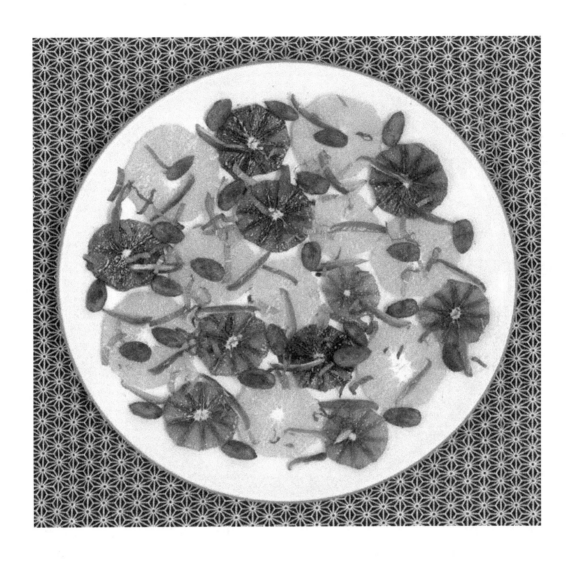

Walnut and Onion Tartine

A quick, scratch-made crust forms the base for this French-inspired meal!

Ingredients: 4 servings

- 2 cups arugula
- ½ cup coarsely chopped walnuts
- 1/3 cup thinly vertically sliced red onion
- 1 oz thin slices prosciutto, chopped
- 1 teaspoon chopped fresh thyme
- 1 teaspoon fresh lemon juice
- 1 oz Parmesan cheese, shaved
- 5 oz all-purpose flour
- Cooking spray
- 6 tablespoons warm water (100° to 110°)
- 1 ¾ teaspoons dry yeast
- 3 tablespoons olive oil, divided
- ¾ teaspoon sugar
- 5/8 teaspoon kosher salt
- ¼ teaspoon black pepper

Directions:

- Preheat oven to 450° F. Combine warm water, dry yeast, and sugar in a medium bowl. Let stand 5 minutes or until bubbly. Stir in 4 teaspoons oil. Weigh or lightly spoon flour into a dry measuring cup and spoons. Level with a knife. Add flour, ¼ teaspoon salt, and pepper to yeast mixture, stirring until a soft dough forms. Turn dough out onto a lightly floured surface. Knead until smooth and elastic.

• Place dough in a large bowl coated with cooking spray, turning to coat top. Cover and let rise in a warm place (85°), free from drafts, 45 minutes or until doubled in size. Punch dough down. Cover and let rest 5 minutes.

• Coat a ceramic baking dish with 2 teaspoons oil. Press dough into pan. Cover and let rise 30 minutes or until puffy. Sprinkle dough with ¼ teaspoon salt, walnuts, onion, prosciutto, and thyme. Bake at 450° F for 18 minutes or until crust is golden and edges are crisp.

• Place arugula in a bowl. Drizzle with remaining 1 tablespoon oil and lemon juice, tossing to coat. Turn bread out onto a clean work surface, and slice crosswise into 4 rectangles. Top each rectangle with about ½ cup arugula mixture and 1 tablespoon shaved Parmesan cheese. Sprinkle evenly with remaining 1/8 teaspoon salt.

Nutritional info per serving: Calories 347, Fat 19.2g, Carbohydrates 32.5g, Protein 10.8g

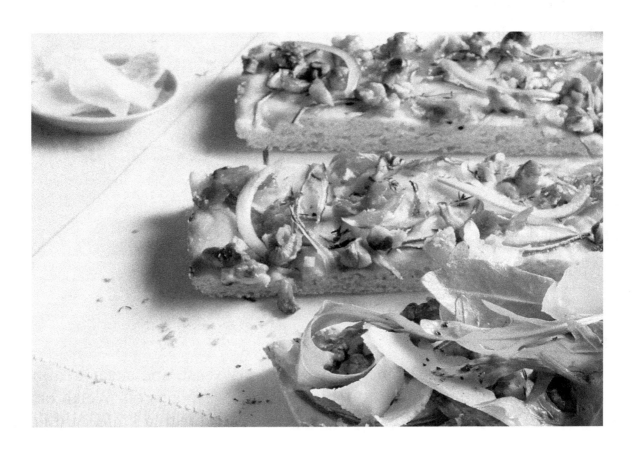

Olives and Avocado Salad with Tomatoes and Feta Cheese

Delicious, colorful and summery avocado salad with black olives, tomatoes and feta cheese!

Ingredients: 6 servings

- 1 jar (5.3 oz) pitted ripe olives without liquid, sliced into thin rounds
- 4 avocados, pitted and diced
- 2 tablespoons capers
- 2 cups grape tomatoes, halved
- 2 cups cubed light feta cheese
- 2 tablespoon extra virgin olive oil
- 1 teaspoon Italian seasoning
- Juice of 2 whole limes
- Pita bread wedges
- Salt and fresh ground pepper, to taste

Directions:

- In a large salad bowl, combine sliced olives, diced avocado, capers, tomatoes, and feta cheese. Set aside.
- In a small mixing bowl whisk together lime juice, extra virgin olive oil, Italian seasoning, and salt and pepper. Whisk until well incorporated.
- Pour dressing over salad and gently toss it all together.
- Serve with pita bread cut into wedges. Enjoy!

Nutritional info per serving: Calories 231, Fat 18.2g, Carbohydrates 10g, Protein 7.2g

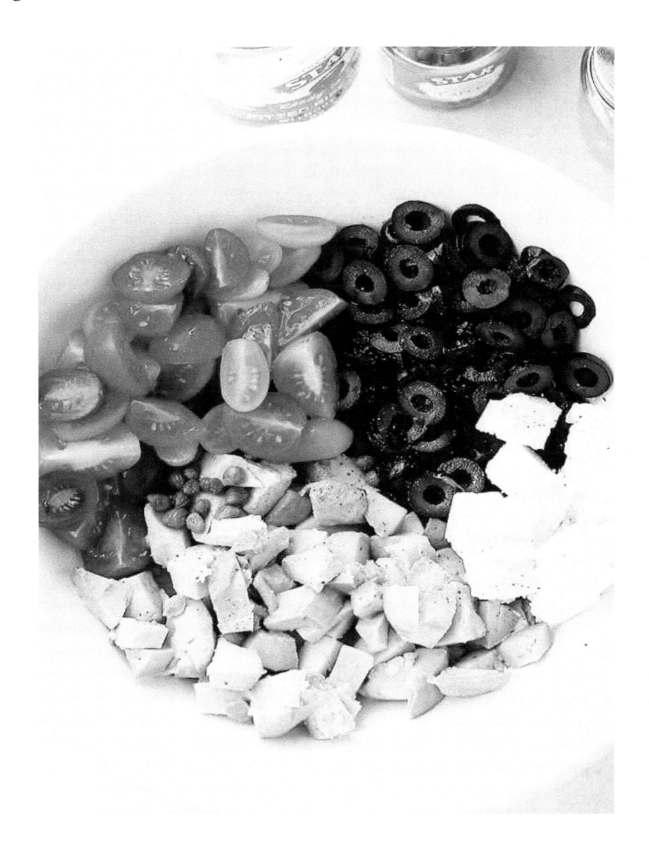

Crispy Artichoke Hearts with Horseradish Sauce

The artichoke hearts are crispy and seasoned, but when you dip them into the horseradish sauce it's really a flavor explosion in your mouth!

Ingredients: 2 servings

- 3 cups frozen artichoke hearts (1-12 oz bag)
- 1 tablespoon lemon juice, fresh squeezed
- 2 tablespoons olive oil
- ½ teaspoon seasoned salt
- ¼ teaspoon ground black pepper

Horseradish Sauce:

- ¼ cup prepared horseradish
- ½ cup mayonnaise
- 1 pinch sea salt
- 1 pinch black pepper

Instructions:

- Combine all the ingredients together and mix well. Chill at least 30 minutes before serving.

Directions:

- Preheat oven to 425° F. Line a cookie sheet with parchment paper.
- Open the bag of frozen artichoke hearts. Drizzle in olive oil and lemon juice, shake to coat hearts well. Sprinkle with seasoned salt and black pepper, tossing again to mix.

- Arrange seasoned artichoke hearts in a single layer on a parchment lined cookie sheet and bake in the middle of the oven at 425° F for 45 minutes, stirring several times during baking, until lightly brown.

- Remove from oven, hearts will crisp up further as they cool. Transfer to a plate and serve with chilled horseradish sauce as a dip.

Nutritional info per serving: Calories 277, Fat 18g, Carbohydrates 26g, Protein 8.8g

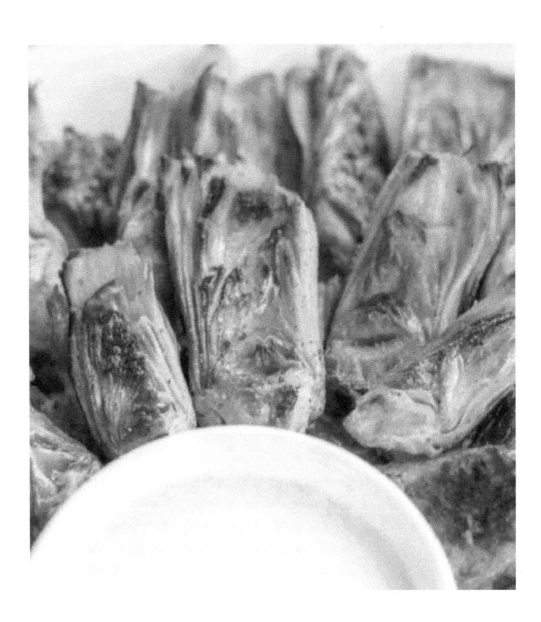

Main Meals

Buckwheat & Asparagus Risotto

A light and delicious buckwheat risotto that won't leave you feeling weighed down!

Ingredients: 4 servings
- 1 ½ cups buckwheat, soaked overnight, drained and rinsed
- 1 big bunch asparagus, chopped into two and tough end discarded
- ¾ cup peas, fresh or thawed frozen
- 1 cup vegetable stock
- Large handful spinach, finely chopped
- 2 tablespoons macadamia, coconut, or olive oil, divided
- 1 small white onion, finely chopped
- 1 lemon, juiced and zested
- 1 tablespoon apple cider vinegar
- 1 tablespoon dried Italian herbs
- 2 cloves garlic, minced
- Handful of parsley, oregano, and basil, roughly chopped plus more for topping
- 2 tablespoons nutritional yeast
- Extra virgin olive oil, for drizzling
- Salt and pepper

Directions:

- Bring the vegetable stock to a boil in a saucepan, then reduce to a simmer.

- In a large pan, heat 1 tablespoon oil and gently fry your asparagus on medium heat, until tender, about 1 minute. Remove from the pan and set aside.

- In the same pan, add remaining oil along with the onion and garlic and cook until soft, about 5 minutes. Add the buckwheat, dried herbs, apple cider vinegar, and lemon juice to the pan and stir so everything is nicely coated.

- Add in the vegetable stock a little bit at a time, stirring frequently. You want the buckwheat to absorb all the liquid slowly and gently.

- Once the buckwheat is almost fully cooked, about 10 minutes, stir in the peas and spinach. Cook for another few minutes, then take off the heat. Stir in the herbs, lemon zest, nutritional yeast, salt and pepper. Taste and adjust seasoning.

- To serve simply spoon into a bowl, top with the asparagus, drizzle some olive oil, and sprinkle some herbs. Enjoy!

Nutritional info per serving: Calories 503, Fat 19g, Carbohydrates 68g, Protein 10g

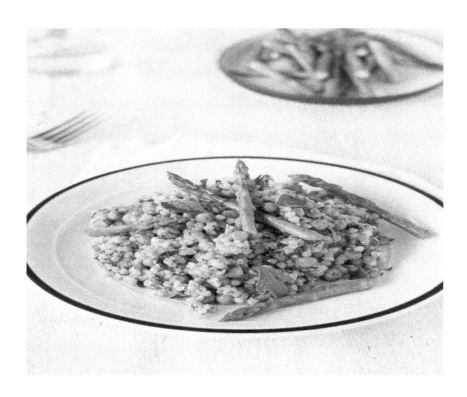

Foil Baked Salmon

This is one of the easiest way to make salmon in foil! It's baked over a bed of asparagus!

Ingredients: 2 servings

- 2 salmon fillets
- 16 asparagus spears
- 1 teaspoon dried oregano
- 2 slices onion
- 1 teaspoon fresh parsley, chopped
- 4 slices lemon
- 1 tablespoon extra virgin olive oil
- Salt
- Ground fresh black pepper

Directions:

- Preheat oven to 400° F. In a medium bowl, place the 2 pieces of salmon. Pour 1 tablespoon olive oil and sprinkle salt, pepper, and dried oregano.
- Cut 2 sheets of foil. It has to be big enough to wrap the salmon and asparagus.
- First place asparagus, about 8 spears, on the sheet of foil.
- Layer fillets over asparagus, then top each with about 2 onion slices and 2 lemon slices.
- Wrap sides of foil inward over salmon, then fold on top and bottom of foil to enclose.
- Place foil packets in a single layer on a baking sheet.

- Bake in preheated oven for about 12-15 minutes. The time will depend on the thickness of the salmon.

- Unwrap and using a large spatula, transfer the foil packets to plates. Serve warm!

Nutritional info per serving: Calories 370, Fat 14g, Carbohydrates 9.5g, Protein 34.9g

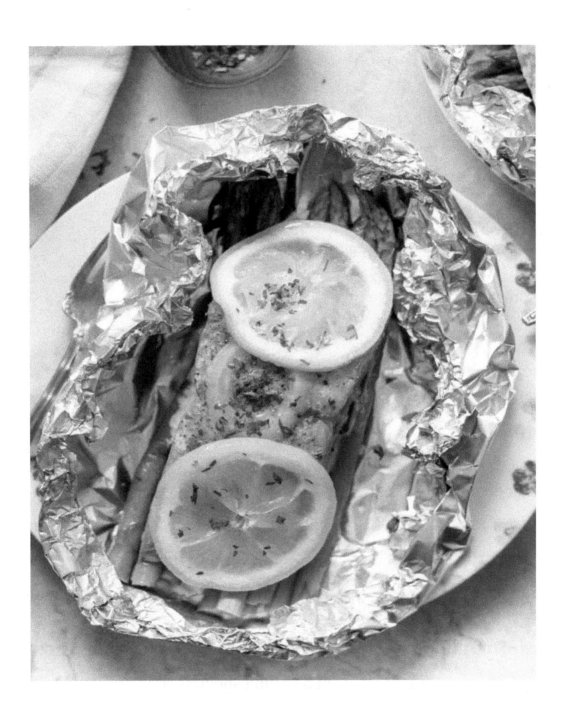

Crispy Chicken with Sweet Chili Rice

Add a bit of spice to your chicken! Enjoy this oriental dish recipe!

Ingredients: 2 servings

- 2 chicken in tempura batter
- ¾ cup white rice
- 2 cups water
- 2 tablespoons sweet chili sauce
- 2 teaspoons coriander
- 2 teaspoons vinegar
- 1 ½ cups white radish

Directions:

- Preheat oven to 450° F. Cook the chicken in the middle of the oven on a baking tray, until crisp and golden, about 15-20 minutes.

- Add rice and water to a medium saucepan and bring to a boil over high heat. Once boiling, lower the heat to a simmer and cover. Ensure it's simmering and not boiling or the rice can cook to quickly. Simmer until water is completely absorbed and rice is tender, about 15-25 minutes. Drain off any excess water if there is any. Let rest for 10 minutes.

- Finely shred the white radish, toss in vinegar and season to taste. Add chili sauce and mix in well.

- Serve on a plate, sprinkle with coriander over radish. Enjoy!

Nutritional info per serving: Calories 472, Fat 12.8g, Carbohydrates 36g, Protein 27g

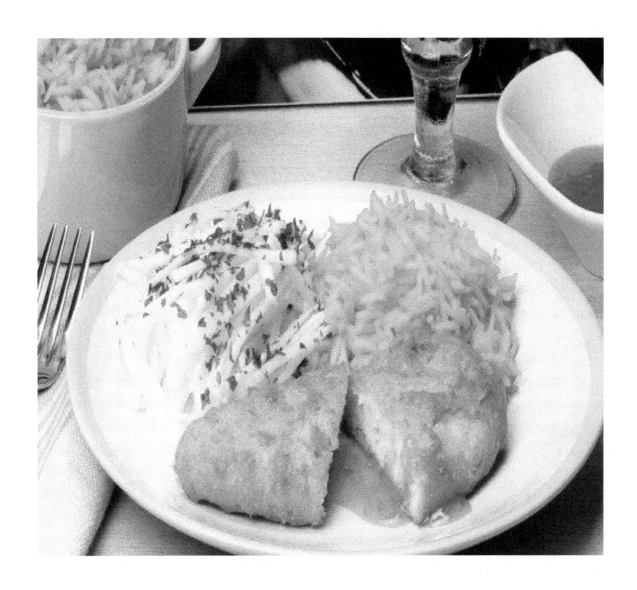

Macaroni & Cheese with Broccoli

This delicious baked macaroni and cheese with broccoli is a healthy make-over of the classic casserole! With its crunchy golden brown breadcrumb topping and uber-creamy cheese sauce you won't miss a thing!

Ingredients: 6 servings

- 3 cups whole-wheat macaroni, uncooked
- 1 large fresh broccoli crown, chopped
- ¼ cup flour
- 2,5 cups milk, divided
- 1 ½ cups shredded extra-sharp cheddar cheese
- 2 teaspoons Dijon mustard
- ¼ teaspoon garlic powder
- ¾ teaspoon paprika
- ¼ teaspoon salt
- 2 teaspoons extra virgin olive oil
- Crumb topping
- Cooking spray
- 3 tablespoons dry breadcrumbs
- ¾ teaspoon salt
- ¼ teaspoon white pepper

Directions:

- Preheat oven to 400° F. Coat a 2-quart baking dish with cooking spray. Bring a large pot of salted water to a boil.

- When water boils cook macaroni 4 minutes. Add the raw fresh broccoli. Continue cooking for 2 minutes longer until the pasta is slightly undercooked; the broccoli should be bright green and crisp tender. Drain thoroughly and return to the pot.

- Meanwhile, prepare cheese sauce. Heat 2 cups milk in a medium saucepan over medium-high heat, stirring often until steaming hot. Whisk together the remaining ½ cup cold milk, flour, Dijon mustard, ¾ teaspoon salt and white pepper in a medium bowl until completely smooth. Whisk the flour mixture into the steaming milk and bring to a simmer whisking often until smooth and thickened. Remove from the heat and stir in the cheese.

- Stir the cheese sauce into the pasta. Transfer the pasta mixture into the prepared baking dish. Stir together breadcrumbs, paprika, ¼ teaspoon salt, and garlic powder in a small bowl. Drizzle in olive oil and stir until completely combined. Sprinkle the crumbs over the pasta and transfer to the oven. Bake until the pasta is bubbling and the topping is golden, 15 to 20 minutes. Enjoy!

Nutritional info per serving: Calories 397, Fat 7.1g, Carbohydrates 59.9g, Protein 20.5g

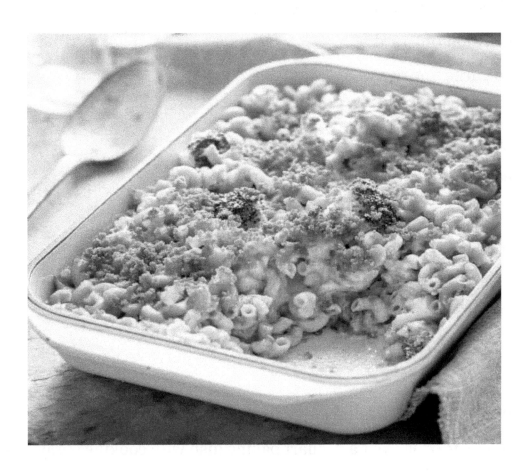

Baked Tofu

This Baked Tofu is super easy to make, and very crispy and delicious!

Ingredients: 2 servings

- 1 block (14 oz) extra-firm tofu, drained
- 1 tablespoon Sriracha
- 2 tablespoons low-sodium soy sauce
- 1 piece ginger, grated
- 2 cloves garlic, grated
- 2 teaspoons rice wine vinegar
- 1 ½ tablespoons cornstarch
- ¼ teaspoon baking powder
- 3 tablespoons toasted sesame oil, divided
- 2 tablespoons packed brown sugar
- Toasted sesame seeds, for garnish
- 1 green onion, thinly sliced, for garnish

Directions:

- Carefully pat tofu dry. On a cutting board, sandwich tofu between doubled layers of paper towels and press down slowly to remove moisture without cracking the block. Remove paper towels and cut tofu into 32 equal pieces. Halve tofu laterally across, then cut the block into a 4x4 grid.

- Make marinade: in a medium bowl, whisk together garlic, ginger, soy sauce, Sriracha, 2 tablespoons sesame oil, vinegar, and sugar until smooth. Set aside half this mixture and reserve for glazing later.

- Preheat oven to 400° F. Meanwhile, add tofu to the bowl and toss gently to coat in marinade. Let sit 15 minutes, then drain off excess marinade.

- In a small bowl, whisk together cornstarch and baking powder. Sprinkle over tofu and gently toss to coat evenly. Drizzle over remaining 1 tablespoon sesame oil and toss to coat each piece.

- Spread tofu evenly out onto a baking sheet and bake for 15 minutes. After 15 minutes, decrease oven temperature to 375° F. Flip tofu pieces to allow for even toasting, then return tray to oven and continue to bake until tofu is crispy on the outside and golden, about 15 minutes more.

- Brush with reserved marinade texture for a glaze finish, then sprinkle with green onions and sesame.

Nutritional info per serving: Calories 158, Fat 6g, Carbohydrates 5g, Protein 14g

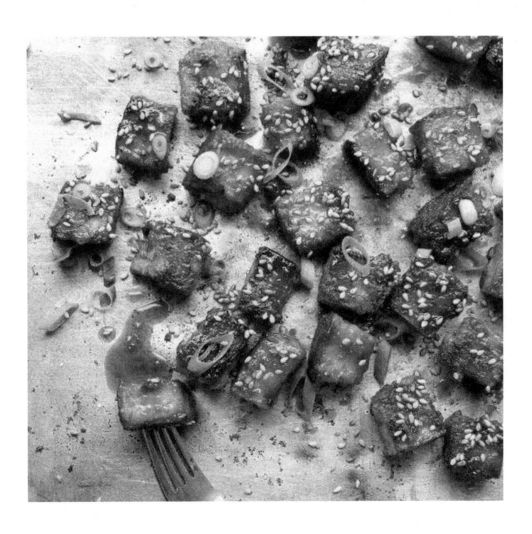

Fish Taco Cabbage Bowl

Fish Taco Cabbage Bowls are a delicious gluten-free, low-glycemic recipe perfect for lunch or dinner!

Ingredients: 4 servings

- 3 large or 4 small fillets of any mild white fish
- 2 teaspoons + 2 teaspoons olive oil
- 1 teaspoon ground cumin
- ½ medium head red cabbage, thinly sliced
- 1 medium head green cabbage, thinly sliced
- 2 teaspoons fish rub of your choice
- ½ teaspoon chili powder
- ½ cup thinly sliced green onion
- Guacamole, for serving

Dressing Ingredients:

- 2 tablespoons fresh-squeezed lime juice
- ½ cup mayonnaise
- 2 teaspoons green tabasco sauce
- Salt to taste

Directions:

- Thaw fish overnight in the refrigerator if frozen.
- Mix the fish rub, ground cumin, and chili powder in a small dish.
- When you're ready to cook, pat fish dry with paper towels, then rub both sides with 2 teaspoons of the olive oil followed by the fish rub mixture.
- Let the fish come to room temperature while you prep the other ingredients.

- Cut away the core of the cabbage and discard, then use a knife or a mandoline slicer to cut the cabbage into thin slices.

- Thinly slice the green onion.

- Whisk together the mayonnaise, lime juice, green tabasco sauce and salt to make the dressing.

- Brush a stove-top grill pan or heavy frying pan with the other 2 tablespoons olive oil and heat the pan about a minute at medium/high heat. Then add the fish and cook about 4 minutes on the first side.

- Turn gently and cook about 4 minutes more on the other side. Cooking time will depend on how thick your pieces of fish are. Fish should feel barely firm to the touch when it's done.

- While the fish cooks, mix about half the green onions into the cabbage mixture and stir in enough dressing to barely moisten the cabbage.

- When the fish is done, let it coll slightly on a cutting board, then use two forks to shred the fish apart.

- Fill bowl with ¼ of the cabbage mixture and top with desired amount of fish. Drizzle a little more dressing over the top.

- Serve right away, with green onions for garnish and guacamole if desired.

Nutritional info per serving: Calories 752, Fat 65g, Carbohydrates 16g, Protein 31g

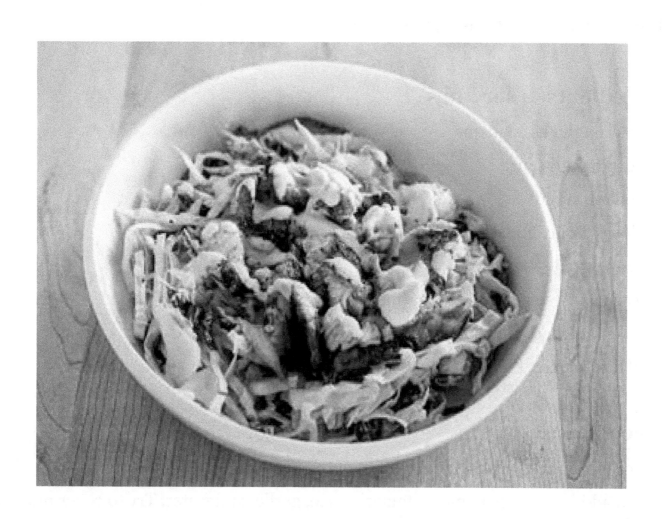

Asian Chicken Thighs

This Asian Chicken Thighs recipe is easy to make and enjoyable to eat! Chicken thighs are very flavorful, and cooking with the skin on will give them a nice flavor boost from the fat.

Ingredients: 4 servings

- 8 chicken thighs, skin on
- ½ cup tamari sauce
- ½ onion, sliced
- 4 cloves garlic, minced
- ¼ cup water
- 1 teaspoon sesame seeds, for garnish
- 1 green onion, chopped for garnish
- Salt and pepper, to taste

Directions:

- Place the chicken thighs at the bottom of the pot.
- Then add in the sliced onions, tamari sauce, garlic, and water. Try to cover most of the chicken in the sauce.
- Set on low heat for 6 hours.
- Season with salt and pepper to taste.
- Garnish with chopped green onions and sesame seeds.
- Roast the thighs in the oven on a baking tray for 15-20 minutes to brown and crisp up the skin.

Nutritional info per serving: Calories 434, Fat 23g, Carbohydrates 5g, Protein 32g

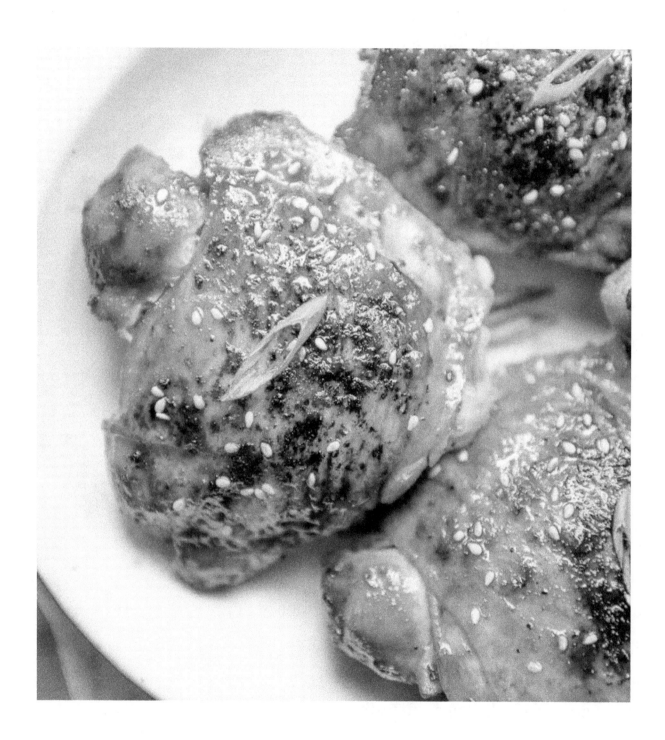

Roast Quail with Rosemary, Thyme and Garlic

Such a simple dish, yet impressive! A few quails seasoned with herb butter and roast in the oven. That's all it takes to put a stunning main course on the table.

Ingredients: 4 servings

- 8 whole quail, washed, dried with paper towel
- 2 fresh thyme sprigs, leaves picked
- 8 cloves garlic, peeled and bruised
- 2 tablespoons butter, cubed
- 1 small lemon, cut into eighths
- 1 fresh rosemary sprig, leaves picked
- ½ cup chicken stock
- Steamed waxy potatoes, to serve
- ¼ cup dry white wine
- Green beans, to serve
- Salt and ground black pepper, to taste

Herb Butter:

- 3 tablespoons butter, at room temperature
- 1 tablespoon fresh rosemary leaves, finely chopped
- 2 tablespoons fresh thyme leaves, finely chopped
- 2 large cloves garlic, crushed
- Salt and ground black pepper, to taste

Directions:

- Preheat the oven to 390° F.

- To make the herb butter, place the butter, thyme, garlic, rosemary, salt and pepper in a small bowl and mix well to combine.

- Use your fingers to carefully loosen the skin over the quail breasts. Spread herb butter over the breasts and then re-cover with the skin.

- Divide the lemon, butter, thyme, garlic and rosemary among the cavities of the quail. Tie the legs together with wet unwaxed string.

- Place the quail in a single layer in a large roasting pan. Roast in preheated oven for 35 minutes or until the juices are pale pink when a fine skewer is inserted into the thigh. Remove the quail from the roasting pan and place on a large plate. Cover loosely with foil and stand for 10 minutes to rest.

- Meanwhile, place roasting pan over medium heat. Add the stock and white wine and cook for 1 minute, scraping with a wooden spoon to dislodge any residue left on the base of the pan. Bring to a boil and simmer, uncovered, for 2-3 minutes or until reduced by ½. Taste and season with salt and pepper.

- Serve the quail with the sauce, potatoes and beans.

Nutritional info per serving: Calories 1084, Fat 26g, Carbohydrates 7g, Protein 14g

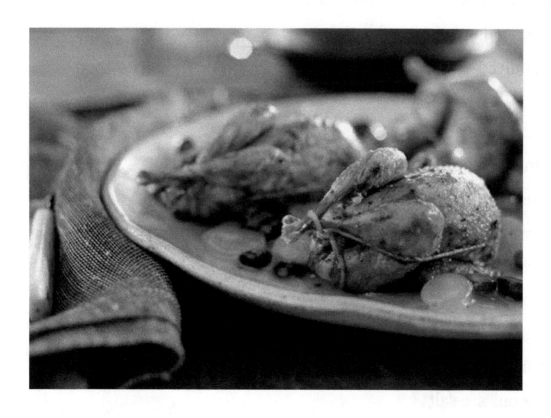

Garlic Butter Roast Turkey

Garlic butter roast turkey cooks up tender, juicy and perfect for your Thanksgiving or any Christmas holiday dinner table!

Ingredients: 10 servings

- One 12-14 pound whole turkey, giblets and neck removed, rinsed and patted dry
- 6 fresh sage leaves, divided
- 2 fresh rosemary sprigs
- 5 fresh thyme sprigs, divided
- 3 medium onions, cut into wedges
- 4 celery ribs, cut into 2 inch pieces
- 5 medium carrots, cut into 2 inch pieces
- 4 cups low-sodium chicken broth
- 1 lemon, halved

Garlic Herb Butter:

- ¾ cup unsalted butter, at room temperature
- 1 ½ tablespoons fresh sage, chopped
- 1 ½ tablespoons fresh rosemary, chopped
- 1 ½ tablespoons fresh thyme leaves, chopped
- 1 tablespoon fresh parsley, chopped
- 5 cloves garlic, minced
- 1 teaspoon black pepper
- 2-3 teaspoons sea salt

Directions:

- If your turkey is frozen, allow 2 to 3 days for it to fully defrost in the refrigerator. Remove giblets and neck, rinse and pat dry.

- To make the butter: In a medium bowl, combine butter, rosemary, sage, parsley, thyme, garlic, salt, and black pepper and stir together until smooth and combined.

- Carefully loosen the skin from the turkey breast with your hands lifting and separating the meat. Do the same for the neck as well as the thighs and legs. Gently rub half of the butter under the skin using your hands and fingers and place 3 sage leaves and 2 thyme sprigs under the skin. Tie the legs together and tuck the wings underneath the turkey, using small skewers to secure, if necessary.

- Place 1/3 of the onions, celery carrots, 2 sage leaves, 2 thyme sprigs, 1 rosemary sprig and lemon halves inside the cavity of the turkey. Place turkey, breast side up in a large roasting pan. Melt the remaining butter in the microwave and brush an even layer over the skin of the turkey. Arrange remaining carrots, celery and herbs in the pan around the turkey. Pour chicken broth to the bottom of the pan.

- Preheat the oven to 425° F and position rack on lower third of the oven. Once the oven is ready, place the roasting pan in the oven and cook for 45 minutes. After 45 minutes, reduce the oven temperature to 350° F and continue to roast until a meat thermometer reads 180° F and juices in the thigh run clear when pierced with a fork, about 2 to 2 ½ hours (or longer depending on your oven), basting with pan broth and drippings every 30 minutes. Cover loosely with foil if turkey browns too quickly. Remove turkey from the pan, place onto a baking sheet, and let rest for 15 minutes before carving. Strain and reserve pan juices for gravy, if desired, and discard vegetables.

Nutritional info per serving: Calories 270, Fat 14g, Carbohydrates 4g, Protein 10g

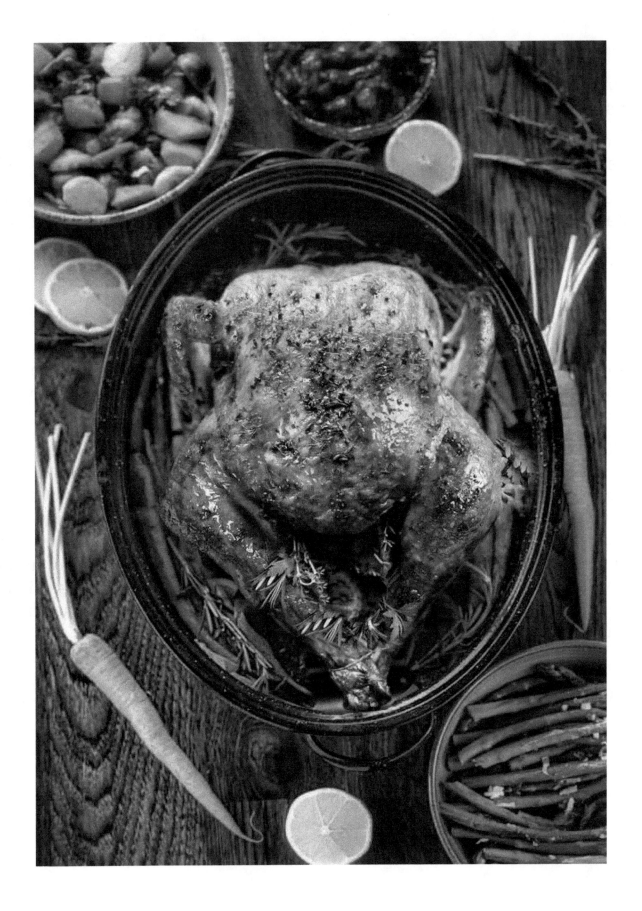

Baked Lemon Butter Tilapia

One of the easiest, most effortless 20 minutes meal ever from start to finish. And it's all made in a single pan!

Ingredients: 4 servings

- 4 tilapia fillets
- ¼ cup unsalted butter, melted
- 3 cloves garlic, minced
- 2 tablespoons freshly squeezed lemon juice to taste
- Zest of 1 lemon
- 2 tablespoons chopped fresh parsley leaves
- Kosher salt and freshly ground black pepper to taste

Directions:

- Preheat the oven to 425° F. Lightly oil a 9x13 baking dish or coat with nonstick spray.
- In a small bowl, whisk together butter, lemon juice, garlic and lemon zest. Set aside.
- Season tilapia with salt and pepper, to taste and place onto the prepared baking dish. Drizzle with butter mixture.
- Place into the oven and bake until fish flakes easily with a fork, about 10-12 minutes.
- Serve immediately, garnished with parsley, if desired.

Nutritional info per serving: Calories 276, Fat 14.5g, Carbohydrates 2.8g, Protein 35.5g

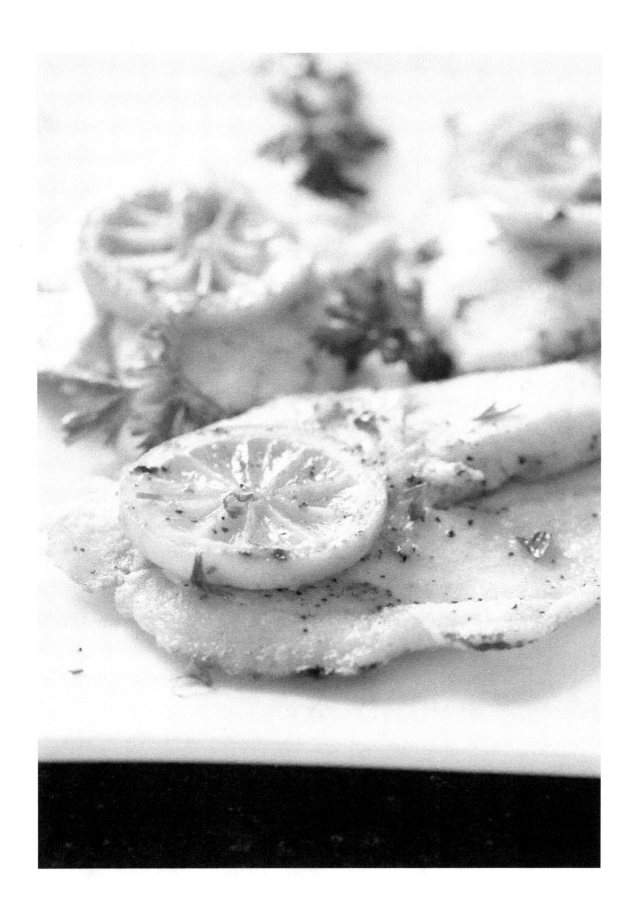

Fried Sardines with Olives

Feeling adventurous? This five-minute fried sardines recipe with olives may be just the ticket to your new favorite unorthodox snack!

Ingredients: 1 serving

- 3 ½ oz sardines in olive oil
- 5 black olives, diced
- 1 tablespoon olive oil
- 1 tablespoon garlic flakes
- 1 teaspoon parsley flakes

Directions:

- Add 1 tablespoon of olive oil to the frying pan and fry everything together for 5 minutes.
- Serve immediately and enjoy!

Nutritional info per serving: Calories 416, Fat 29g, Carbohydrates 5g, Protein 21g

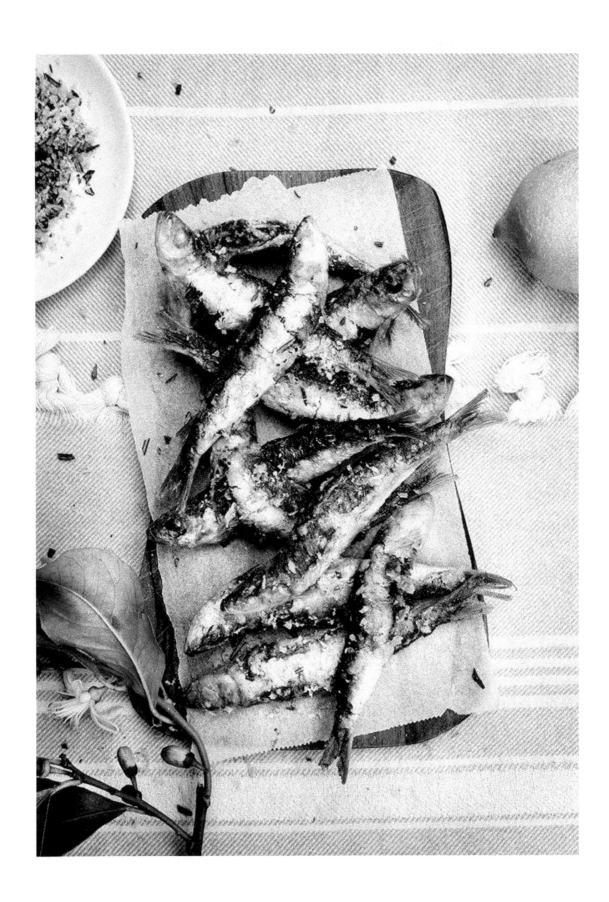

Salmon Curry

Curries are a really easy and delicious meal you can make even when you have little cooking experience. Plus, you can vary them a lot by using different vegetables.

Ingredients: 2 servings

- 1 lb of raw salmon, diced
- ½ medium onion, finely chopped
- 1 ½ tablespoons curry powder
- 1 teaspoon garlic powder
- 2 cups green beans, diced
- 2 tablespoons basil, chopped, for garnish
- 2 cups bone broth
- Cream from the top of 1 can of coconut milk
- 2 tablespoons coconut oil
- Salt and pepper to taste

Directions:

- Cook the diced onion in the coconut oil until translucent.
- Add in the green beans and saute for a few minutes more.
- Add in the broth or water and bring to a boil.
- Add in the curry powder, garlic powder, and salmon.
- Add in the coconut cream and simmer until the salmon is cooked, about 3-5 minutes.
- Add salt and pepper to taste and serve with the chopped basil.

Nutritional info per serving: Calories 621, Fat 41g, Carbohydrates 11g, Protein 45g

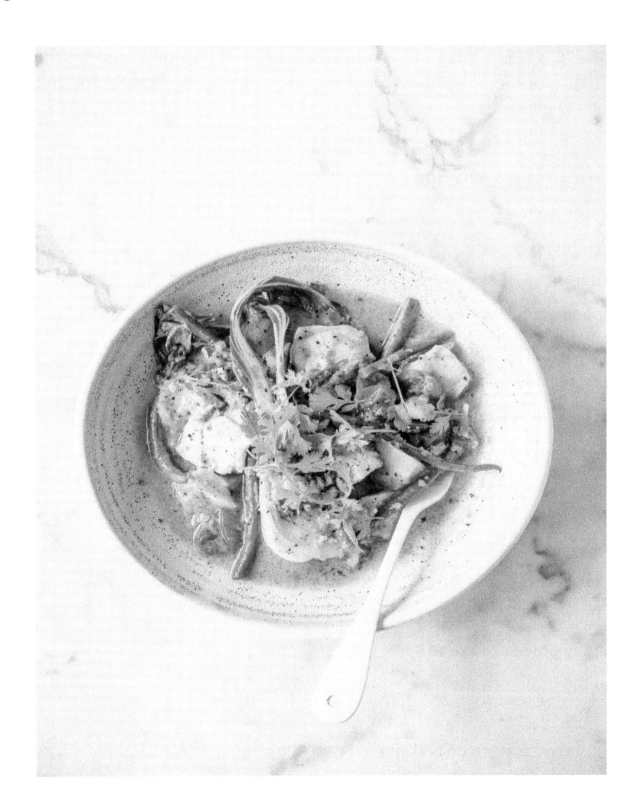

Fish Casserole with Mushrooms and French Mustard

So hearty. So satisfying. And so, so simple to make. If you love fish, mushrooms and creamy, rich sauces, be prepared to fall head over heels in love with this amazing casserole!

Ingredients: 6 servings

- 25 oz white fish
- 15 oz mushrooms
- 3 oz butter
- 20 oz broccoli or cauliflower
- 2 tablespoons fresh parsley
- 8 oz shredded cheese
- 2 tablespoons mustard
- 3 oz butter or olive oil
- 2 cups heavy whipping cream
- 1 teaspoon salt
- Pepper to taste

Directions:

- Preheat the oven to 350° F.
- Cut the mushrooms into wedges. Fry in butter until the mushrooms have softened, about 5 minutes. Add salt, pepper, and parsley.
- Pour in the heavy cream and mustard and lower the heat. Let simmer for 5-10 minutes to reduce the sauce a bit.

- Season the fish with salt and pepper and place in a greased baking dish. Sprinkle ¾ of the cheese on and pour the creamed mushrooms on top. Top with the remaining cheese.

- Bake for about 30 minutes if the fish is frozen, or slightly less if it's fresh. Probe with a sharp knife after 20 minutes; the fish is done if it flakes easily with a fork. And remember that the fish will continue to cook even after you have taken it out of the oven.

- Meanwhile, make the side dish. Cut the broccoli or cauliflower into florets. Boil in lightly salted water for a few minutes. Strain off the water and add olive oil or butter.

- Mash coarsely with a wooden spoon or fork.

- Season with salt and pepper and serve with the fish.

Nutritional info per serving: Calories 528, Fat 41g, Carbohydrates 10g, Protein 35g

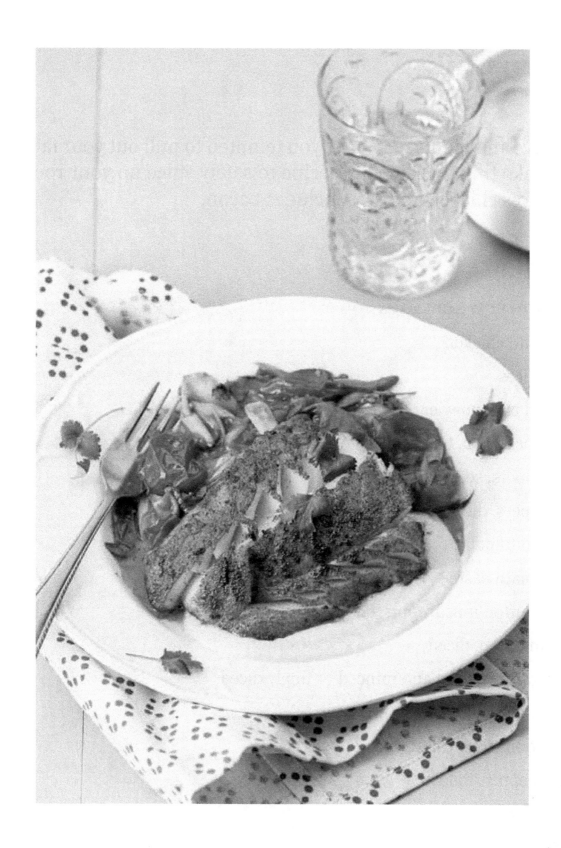

Chicken Chili

Colder days and nights may have you tempted to pull out your favorite chili recipe. Make this chicken chili recipe to safely spice up your routine! This chili features chicken and also includes bacon.

Ingredients: 6 servings

- 2 lbs ground chicken
- 4 bacon slices
- 1 teaspoon chili powder
- ¼ cup avocado oil, to cook with
- 3 chili peppers, seeds removed and finely diced
- 2 bell peppers, diced
- 1 can diced tomatoes
- ½ can tomato paste
- 10 white button mushrooms, chopped
- 1 medium onion, diced
- 2 cloves garlic, peeled and minced or finely diced
- 2 tablespoons Italian seasoning
- 2 tablespoons fresh cilantro, chopped
- Salt and pepper, to taste

Directions:

- Add the avocado oil to a large pot over medium/high heat. Add the ground chicken, diced bacon, and diced onion and sautè until browned, about 5 to 6 minutes.

- Add the bell peppers, mushrooms, and chili peppers to the pot and sauté for about 5 minutes. Season with salt and pepper, to taste.

- Add the diced tomatoes, tomato paste, Italian seasoning, and chili powder to the pot. Cover and cook for 50 minutes, stirring occasionally.

- Remove the lid and add the garlic and fresh cilantro to the pot. Continue to cook, uncovered, for about 10 minutes. Season with additional salt pepper, to taste.

Nutritional info per serving: Calories 398, Fat 25g, Carbohydrates 12g, Protein 26g

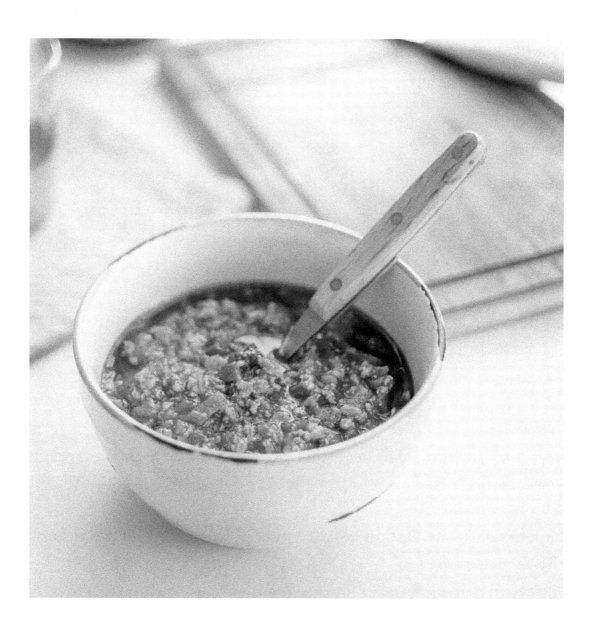

Garlic & Rosemary Grilled Lamb Chops

Grilled lamb chops infused with rosemary and garlic flavors! This delicious dish is super easy to make!

Ingredients: 4 servings

- 2 pounds lamb loin
- 4 cloves garlic, minced
- 1 tablespoon fresh rosemary, chopped
- ¼ cup olive oil
- Zest of 1 lemon
- ½ teaspoon ground black pepper
- 1 ¼ teaspoon kosher salt

Directions:

- Combine the garlic, rosemary, lemon zest, olive oil, salt and pepper in a measuring cup.
- Pour the marinade over the lamb chops, making sure to flip them over to cover them completely. Cover and marinate the chops in the fridge for as little as 1 hour, or as long as overnight.
- Heat the grill to medium/high heat, then sear the lamb chops for 2-3 minutes, on each side. Lower the heat to medium then cook them for 5-6 minutes, or until the internal temperature reads 150 degrees F.
- Allow the lamb chops to rest on a plate covered with aluminum foil for 5 minutes before serving.

Nutritional info per serving: Calories 272, Fat 7.8g, Carbohydrates 1.2g, Protein 23.2g

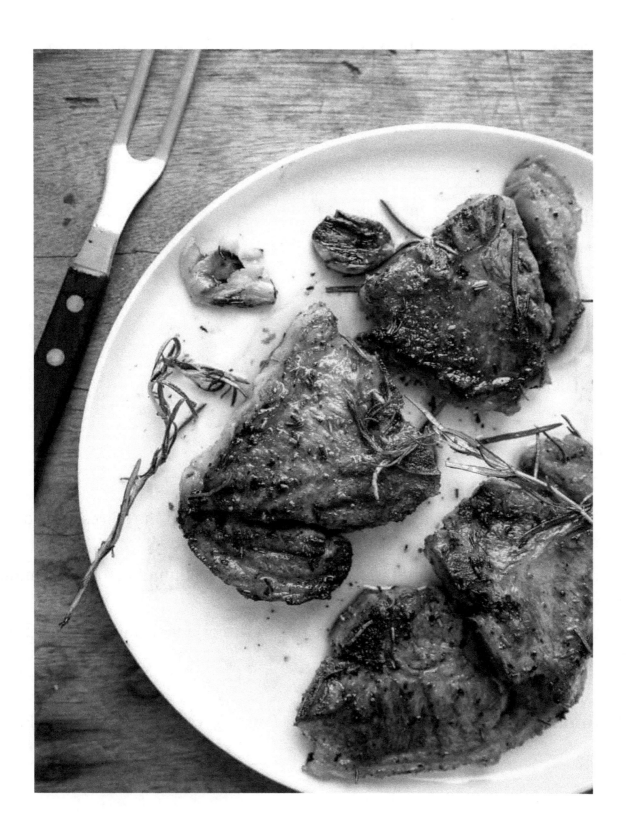

Indian Spiced Cauliflower Rice

This Indian spiced cauliflower rice is a quick, easy and wonderfully nutritious alternative to regular rice!

Ingredients: 4 servings

- 1 cauliflower, leaves and stalk removed
- 1 tablespoon coconut oil
- 1 teaspoon turmeric
- 1 teaspoon cumin
- 2 tablespoons fresh coriander, chopped roughly
- Salt and pepper to taste

Directions:

- Start by finely chopping the cauliflower.
- Heat the oil gently in a frying pan for 30 seconds, then add the spices and cook for another 30 seconds.
- Add the finely chopped cauliflower and stir fry over medium heat for 3-5 minutes until cooked to your liking.
- Stir through some salt and pepper and the fresh coriander and serve with your favorite curry.

Nutritional info per serving: Calories 64, Fat 3.5g, Carbohydrates 4.3g, Protein 3g

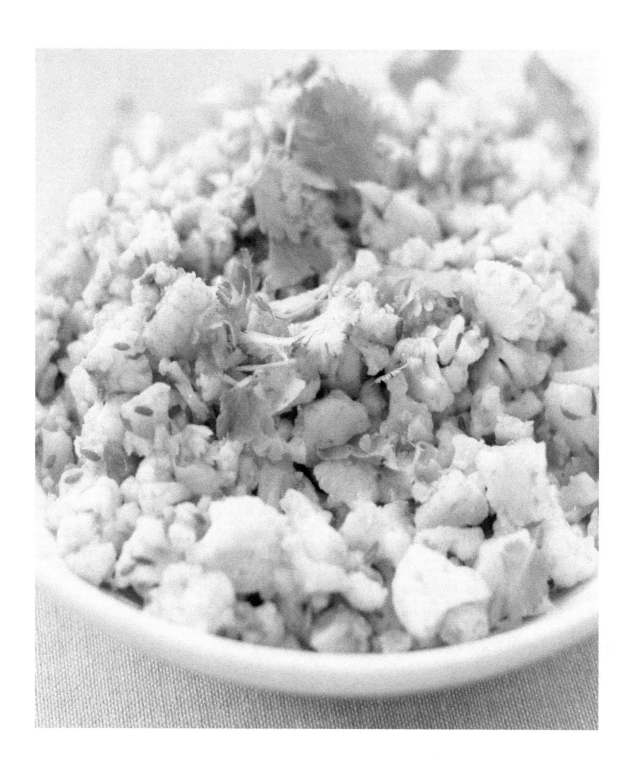

Cheesy Asparagus

This baked cheesy asparagus recipe needs just 5 ingredients and is ready in 20 minutes. The perfect easy, healthy dish!

Ingredients: 4 servings

- 1 lb asparagus, trimmed
- 2 tablespoons olive oil
- ½ cup Parmesan cheese, shredded
- ½ cup mozzarella cheese, shredded
- 1 tablespoon Italian seasoning
- Black pepper
- Sea salt

Directions:

- Preheat the oven to 400° F. Line a baking sheet with foil or parchment paper.
- Toss the asparagus with olive oil, sea salt, black pepper, and half of the Italian seasoning. Arrange in a single layer on the lined baking sheet.
- Roast in the oven for about 7-9 minutes, until the asparagus is bright green and just starting to soften.
- Mix together the mozzarella and Parmesan cheese, then sprinkle over the asparagus. Top with remaining Italian seasoning.
- Return to the oven for another 6-8 minutes, until the cheese is melted and golden.

Nutritional info per serving: Calories 160, Fat 12g, Carbohydrates 3g, Protein 8g

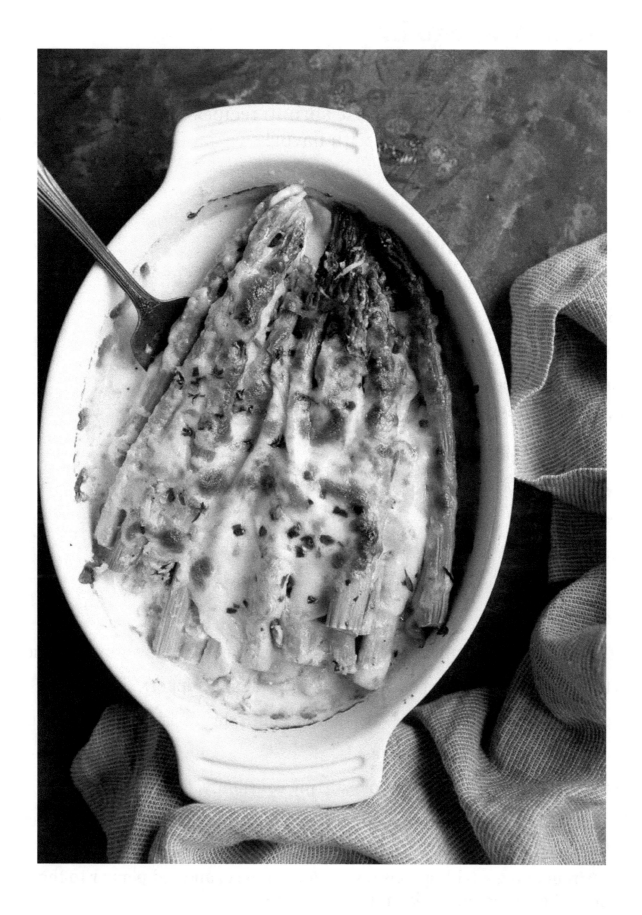

Garlic Butter Shrimp

Garlic butter shrimp is one of those shrimp recipes that you'll make again and again, so easy and bursting with flavor!

Ingredients: 4 servings

- 1 pound shrimp, peeled and deveined
- 6 tablespoons butter, divided
- 5 cloves garlic, minced
- ½ cup chicken stock
- 2 tablespoons parsley, minced
- 2 tablespoons lemon juice
- ¼ teaspoon red pepper flakes
- ½ teaspoon black pepper
- ½ teaspoon kosher salt

Directions:

- Heat 2 tablespoons of butter in a large heavy bottomed skillet over medium heat.
- Add the shrimp to the skillet and sprinkle with salt and pepper.
- Cook, stirring occasionally, for 4-5 minutes or until shrimp is cooked through.
- Remove shrimp to a plate and set aside.
- Add the garlic to the skillet and cook, stirring constantly, for 30 seconds.
- Add the chicken stock and whisk to combine. Simmer until stock has reduced by half, about 5-10 minutes.
- Add the remaining 4 tablespoons butter, lemon juice, and red pepper to the sauce. Stir to melt the butter and cook for 2 more minutes.

- Remove from heat and return the shrimp to the sauce. Sprinkle the parsley over the top and stir to combine.
- Serve immediately.

Nutritional info per serving: Calories 307, Fat 18g, Carbohydrates 7g, Protein 27g

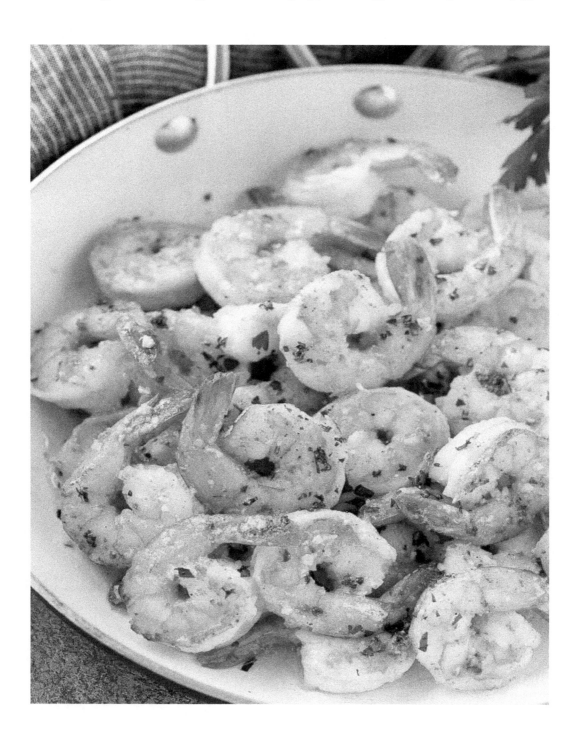

Ground Beef & Broccoli

A one-skillet wonder! Real food, affordable ingredients, simple prep, tasty dinner, and easy clean up. It's fast food, made right in your kitchen!

Ingredients: 2 servings

- 10 oz ground beef
- 9 oz broccoli
- 3 oz butter
- ½ cup mayonnaise or crème fraîche
- Salt and pepper, to taste

Directions:

- Rinse and trim the broccoli, including the stem. Cut into small florets. Peel the stem and cut into small pieces.
- Heat up a hearty dollop of butter in a frying pan where you can fit both the ground beef and broccoli.
- Brown the ground beef on high heat until it's almost done. Season with salt and pepper to taste.
- Lower the heat. Add more butter and fry the broccoli for 3-5 minutes. Stir the ground beef every now and then.
- Season the broccoli. Top with the remaining butter and serve while still hot. It's also delicious to serve with an extra dollop of crème fraîche or mayonnaise.

Nutritional info per serving: Calories 518, Fat 34g, Carbohydrates 9g, Protein 31g

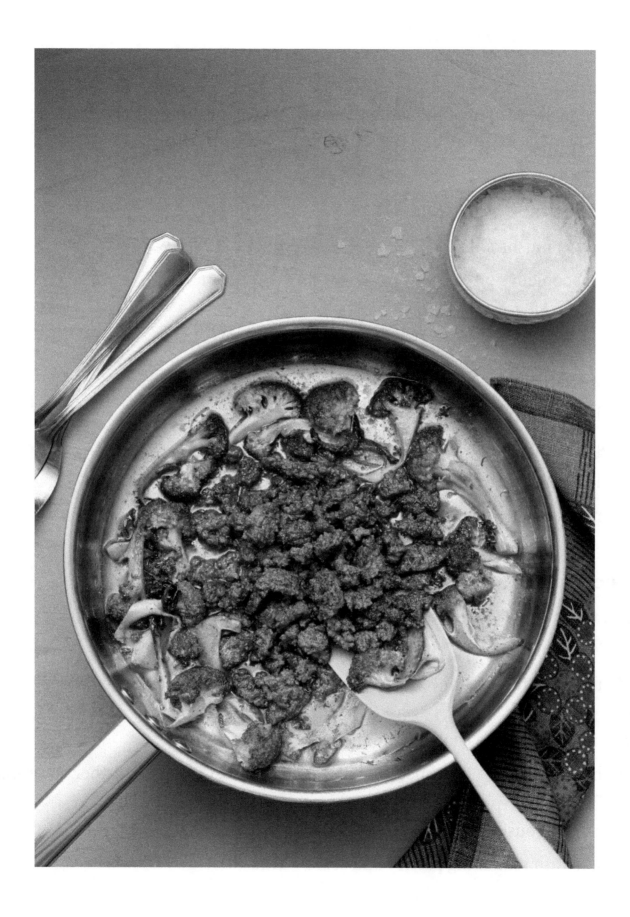

Garlic Mushrooms

Buttery garlic mushrooms with a mouth watering herb garlic butter sauce! You'll love this 10-minutes dish that goes with anything!

Ingredients: 4 servings

- 1 lb button mushrooms
- 1 tablespoon olive oil
- 4 tablespoons unsalted butter
- ½ onion, chopped
- 4 cloves garlic, minced
- 2 tablespoons chopped fresh parsley
- 1 teaspoon fresh thyme leaves, chopped
- 2 tablespoons dry white wine
- Salt and pepper to taste

Directions:

- Heat the butter and oil in a large pan or skillet over medium/high heat.
- Sautè the onion until softened, about 3 minutes.
- Add the mushrooms and cook for about 4-5 minutes until golden and crispy on the edges.
- Pour in the wine and cook for 2 minutes, to reduce slightly.
- Stir through thyme, 1 tablespoon of parsley and garlic. Cook for a further 30 seconds, until fragrant.
- Season generously with salt and pepper.
- Sprinkle with remaining parsley and serve warm.

Nutritional info per serving: Calories 168, Fat 11g, Carbohydrates 5g, Protein 4g

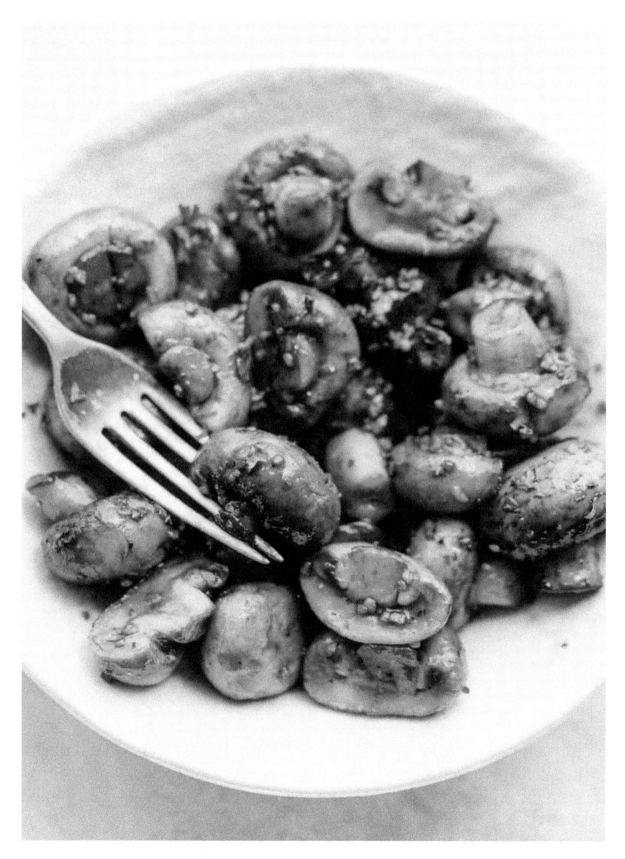

Appetizers & Snacks

Broccoli Cheddar Bites

Cheesy baked broccoli snacks, great for a brunch, kid-friendly lunch, or party!

Ingredients: 24 bites

- 1 large bunch of broccoli florets
- ½ cup, packed, torn fresh bread
- 2 eggs, lightly beaten
- ¼ cup mayonnaise
- ¼ cup grated onion
- 1 ½ teaspoons lemon zest
- 1 cup, packed, grated sharp cheddar cheese
- ¼ teaspoon freshly ground black pepper
- ½ teaspoon kosher salt

Directions:

- Place 1 inch of water in a pot with a steamer basket. Bring to a boil. Add the broccoli florets. Steam the broccoli florets for 5 minutes, until just tender. Rinse with cold water to stop the cooking. Finely chop the steamed broccoli florets. You should have 2 to 2 ½ cups.

- Place the beaten eggs and the torn bread in a large bowl. Mix until the bread is completely moistened. Add the grated onion, mayonnaise, cheese, lemon zest, salt and pepper. Stir in the minced broccoli.

- Preheat the oven to 350° F. Coat the wells of 2 mini muffin pans with olive oil. Distribute the broccoli mixture in the muffin wells.

- Bake at 350° F for 25 minutes until cooked through and lightly browned on top. If you don't have mini muffin pans, you can cook the bites freeform. Just grease a baking sheet and spoon large dollops of the mixture onto the pan. Baking time is the same.

Nutritional info per serving: Calories 62, Fat 4.8g, Carbohydrates 3g, Protein 1.7g

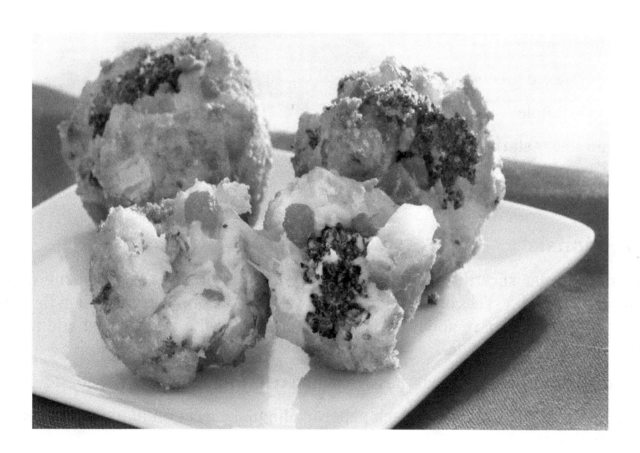

No Bake Zucchini Roll-Ups

Easy no bake zucchini roll ups with guacamole, carrots, celery and mixed greens stuffed in a whole peperoncini! Every bite is so fresh, crunchy and delicious, sometimes you just have to eat on the spot.

Ingredients: 20 roll-ups

- 1 large zucchini
- 1 jar peperoncini
- 1 medium carrot
- Handful mixed greens
- 1 tub guacamole
- 1 single celery stalk
- Fresh dill

Directions:

• Using a peeler slice the zucchini the long way, on all sides to avoid the center. Basically, make 3-4 slices on one side and move on to the opposite side, then the other two sides until you have about 20 slices. Don't discard the middle, just add to your next skillet meal. Set aside.

• Using a mandoline slicer, cut the carrots and celery into thin strips. Set aside.

• Finally, cut the top part off of each peperoncini, make a cut on one side to open and clean seeds out.

Arranging the Roll Ups:

• On a flat surface place one zucchini stip. Spread a dab of guacamole on one end. Place a peperoncini on top of the guacamole, open side up. Fill pocket whole of the peperoncini with guacamole. Add in 1-2 mixed green leaves, 3 strips of carrots, 1-2 strips of celery, fresh dill and roll it tight until you reach the end of the zucchini. If you need help keeping the zucchini roll ups tight in place, add another dab of guacamole on the end part of the zucchini to stick together.

• Do this step until you've used all the ingredients.

• Serve cold and refrigerate leftover for up to 24 hours. The guacamole will darken after this time.

Nutritional info per serving: Calories 214, Fat 4.7g, Carbohydrates 4g, Protein 5g

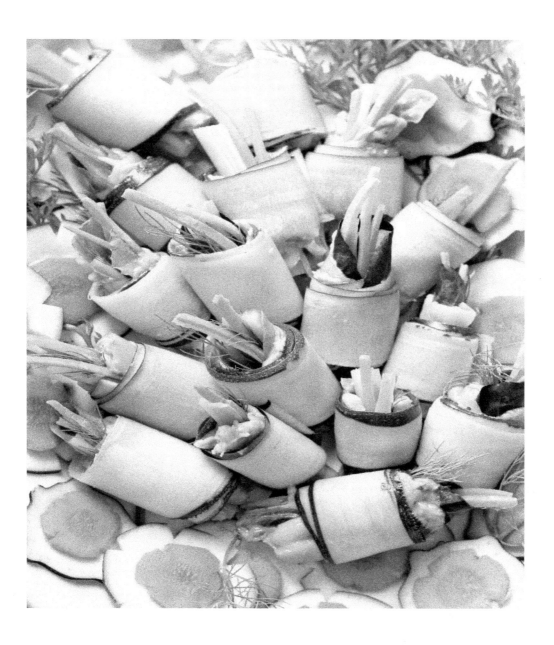

Avocado Deviled Eggs

These avocado deviled eggs are delicious and perfect for the kids. They are full of good fats, from avocado, and protein from the eggs. This makes them a great snack!

Ingredients: 3 servings

- 3 eggs
- 1 avocado
- 1 tablespoon chopped chives
- 1 tablespoon freshly squeezed lime juice

Directions:

- Peel your hard boiled eggs and cut them in half, lengthways.
- Remove the cooked yolk and add to a mixing bowl along with the avocado and lime juice.
- Mash, with a fork, until you achieve the desired texture. Stir in the chopped chives.
- Either spoon the mixture back into the eggs or pipe it into the eggs using a piping bag or zip lock back.
- Serve straight away.

Nutritional info per serving: Calories 156, Fat 5.3g, Carbohydrates 3.8g, Protein 3.4g

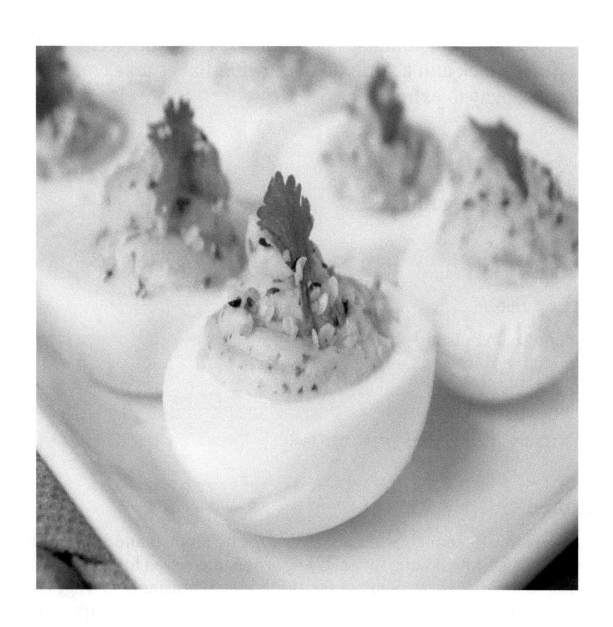

Spicy Deviled Eggs

If you've wondered how to make spicy deviled eggs, this recipe is for you! A spicy sriracha kick and a sprinkle of red chili flakes take creamy deviled eggs from just okay to extraordinary.

Ingredients: 24 egg halves

- 12 large eggs
- 1 tablespoon sriracha sauce
- 1/3 cup mayonnaise
- 1 tablespoon Dijon mustard
- Fine chili flakes
- Fresh chives, minced
- Salt and freshly ground black pepper to taste

Directions:

- Fill a saucepan with enough water to cover eggs by an inch and bring to full boil. Carefully lower eggs into boiling water. Let eggs boil uncovered for about 30 seconds. Reduce heat to low and cover. Simmer for 11 minutes. Transfer boiled eggs to a bowl of ice water. When cool enough to handle, gently break shell apart and peel. If possible, refrigerate eggs overnight, making them easier to cut.

- Once eggs are cool, cut in half lengthwise with a very sharp knife. Carefully spoon yolks out into a small bowl and arrange whites on serving platter.

- In a medium bowl, mash yolks into a paste with the back of a fork. Add mayonnaise, sriracha sauce and mustard; whisk until smooth. Season to taste with salt, freshly ground black pepper and more sriracha if you like.

- Spoon or pipe filling into egg white halves.

- Cover and refrigerate eggs for 2 hours or more (up to 1 day). Once chilled sprinkle generously with fine chili flakes and minced chives. Serve and enjoy!

Nutritional info per serving: Calories 53, Fat 4g, Carbohydrates 0.6g , Protein 2 g

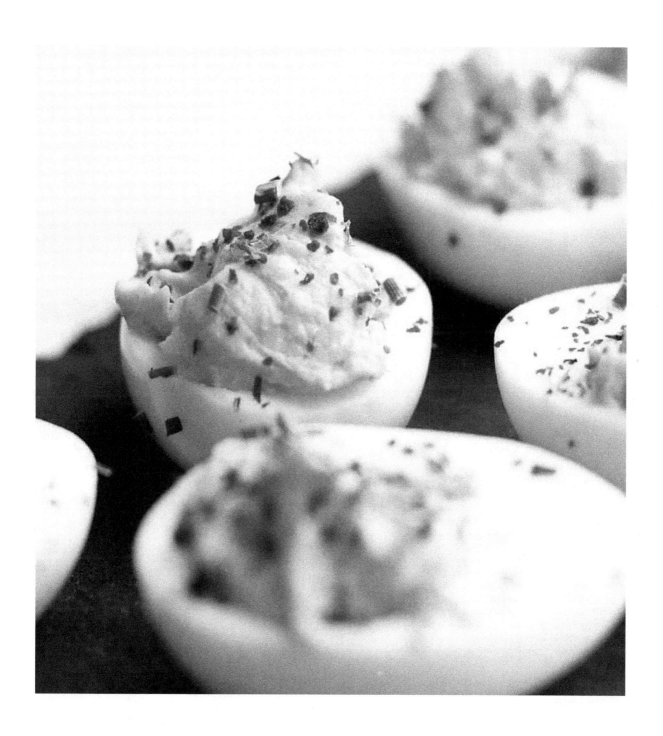

Spicy Roasted Nuts

Crunchy, salty, and spicy! These nuts will keep you and your guests coming back for more, and more, and more!

Ingredients: 6 servings

- 8 oz pecans or almonds or walnuts
- 1 tablespoon olive oil or coconut oil
- 1 teaspoon paprika powder or chili powder
- 1 teaspoon ground cumin
- 1 teaspoon salt

Directions:

- Mix all ingredients in a medium frying pan, and cook on medium heat until the almonds are warmed through.
- Let cool and serve as a snack with a drink. Store in a container with lid at room temperature.

Nutritional info per serving: Calories 201, Fat 7g, Carbohydrates 5g, Protein 4g

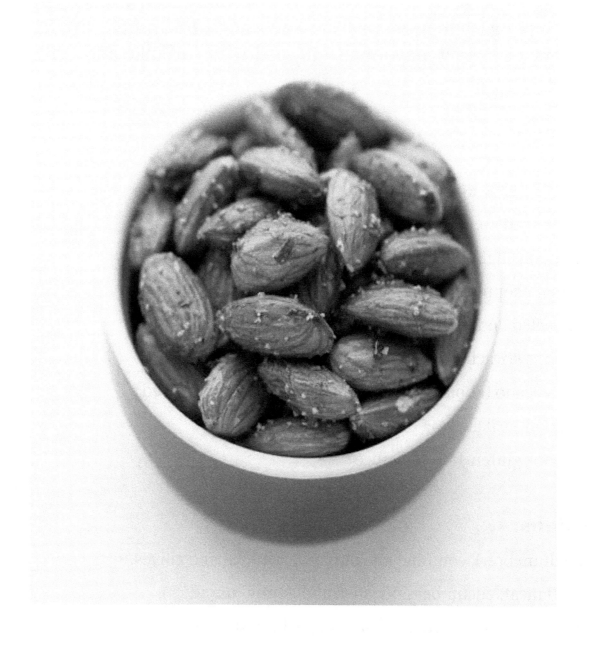

Crab Salad Stuffed Avocado

These crab salad stuffed avocados are a healthy snack or appetizer, and they are super easy to prepare! These avocados are stuffed with lump crab, cucumbers and spicy mayonnaise topped with furikake and drizzled with soy sauce.

Ingredients: 2 servings

- 4 oz lump crab meat
- 2 tablespoons light mayonnaise
- 1 teaspoon chopped fresh chives
- ¼ cup peeled and diced cucumber
- 2 teaspoons sriracha, plus more for drizzling
- 1 small avocado (about 4 oz avocado when pitted and peeled)
- ½ teaspoon furikake
- 2 teaspoons gluten-free soy sauce

Directions:

- In a medium bowl, combine mayonnaise, sriracha and chives.
- Add crab meat, cucumber and chive and gently toss.
- Cut the avocado open, remove pit and peel the skin or spoon the avocado out.
- Fill the avocado halves equally with crab salad.
- Top with furikake and drizzle with soy sauce.

Nutritional info per serving: Calories 194, Fat 13g, Carbohydrates 7g, Protein 12g

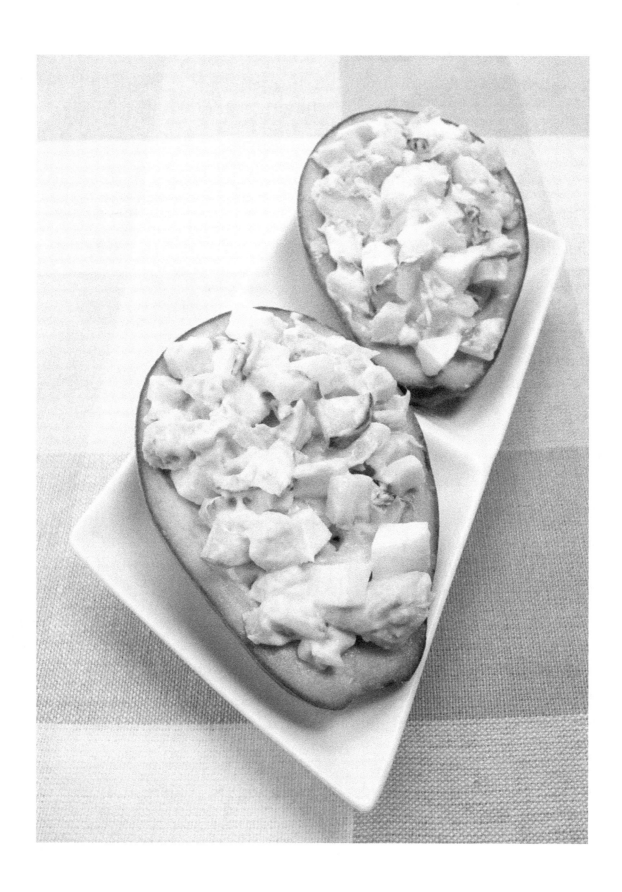

Cheddar Olives

These Cheddar Olives come together in a snap! It's the perfect snack for catching up on your TV watching, or having a good chat!

Ingredients: 6-8 servings

- 1 8-10 jar pitted olives, either pimento-stuffed or plain
- 1 cup all-purpose flour
- 1 ½ cups shredded sharp cheddar cheese
- ¼ teaspoon freshly grated black pepper
- 4 tablespoons unsalted butter, softened

Directions:

- Preheat oven to 400° F. Drain the olives well, and dry them completely with clean dish towels. Set aside.
- Combine the cheese, flour, butter, and spices in a medium bowl and knead it within the bowl until a dough forms. If the dough is still crumbly and won't hold together, add water 1 teaspoon at a time until it does.
- Pinch of a small amount of dough, and press it as thin as you can between your fingers to flatten. Wrap and smoosh the dough around a dry olive. Pinch off any excess, then roll the olive in your hands until smooth. Continue until all the olives are covered.
- Bake for 15-20 minutes, or until golden brown all over. Serve immediately and enjoy!

Nutritional info per serving (8 servings): Calories 195, Fat 12.2g, Carbohydrates 8.1g, Protein 6.9g

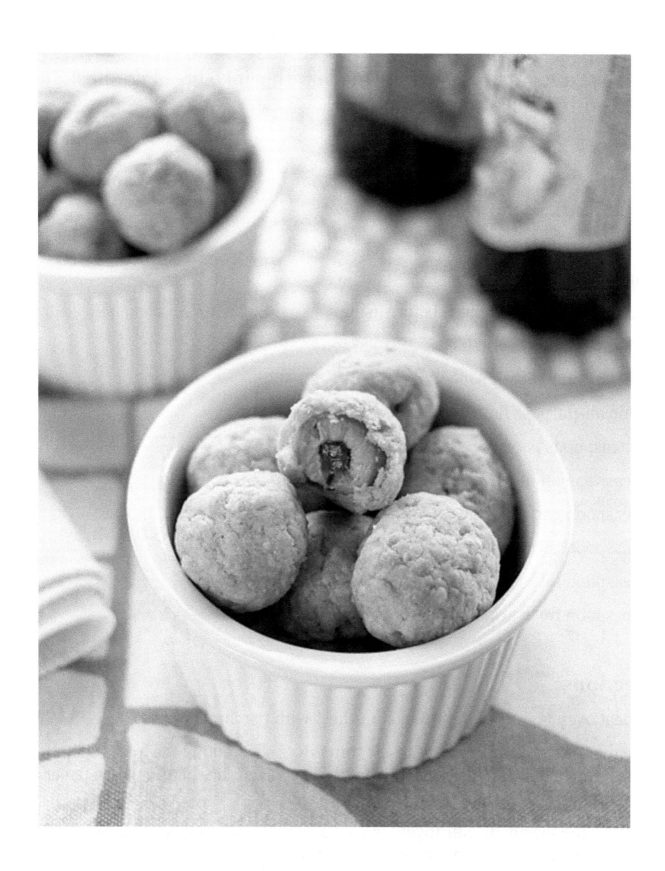

Crispy Breaded Tofu Nuggets

These bite sized tofu nuggets are made with panko bread crumbs! They're perfect with dinner or as an appetizer!

Ingredients: 4 servings

- 1 block extra firm tofu
- 1 cup panko bread crumbs
- 2 flax eggs, let sit 5 minutes before using
- ½ cup vegetable broth
- 1 tablespoon light soy sauce
- ½ cup all-purpose flour
- 1 ½ teaspoons paprika
- ½ teaspoon onion powder
- ½ teaspoon garlic powder
- ½ teaspoon cayenne pepper
- ¼ teaspoon salt
- ¼ teaspoon fresh ground black pepper

Directions:

- Preheat oven to 400° F. Line a baking sheet with parchment paper.

- Slice the tofu into 10 squares. Cut the tofu into 5 slices along the long edge, then cut each column in half to make squares. Lightly press each slice of tofu with a paper towel to remove some of the liquid.

- To make the marinade, stir together the vegetable broth and soy sauce in a shallow pan. Marinate the tofu in the vegetable broth mixture for at least 10 minutes.

- Prepare 3 bowls: one with the flour, one with panko bread crumbs and spices, and one with the flax eggs. Coat the tofu in the flour, then the flax eggs, and finally the panko

- Bake at 400° F on the parchment lined baking sheet for 15 minutes. Carefully flip the tofu bites over, then bake for another 15 minutes. They're ready when golden brown and crispy. Enjoy!

Nutritional info per serving: Calories 127, Fat 6.4g, Carbohydrates 23g, Protein 5g

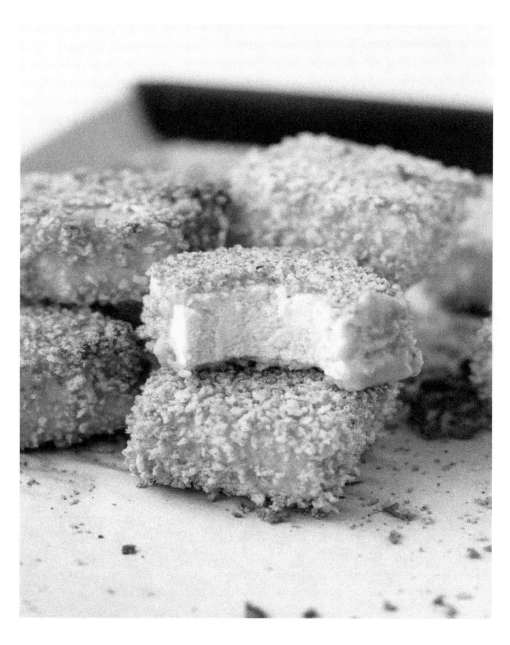

Rosemary Toasted Walnuts

Rosemary Toasted Walnuts are perfect for snacking on! These walnuts are great on salad or enjoyed on their own!

Ingredients: 8 servings

- 2 cups raw walnuts
- 2 tablespoons fresh rosemary, finely chopped
- ¼ cup olive oil
- ½ teaspoon salt
- 1 teaspoon pepper

Directions:

- Preheat oven to 350° F. Line a baking sheet with parchment paper.
- In a bowl, whisk together olive oil, rosemary, salt, and pepper.
- Add in walnuts and toss until completely covered in olive oil mixture.
- Bake the walnuts for 10-15 minutes in the oven, tossing every 4-5 minutes until they're golden brown. The walnuts cook quickly, so be careful not to burn them. Enjoy!

Nutritional info per serving (1/4 cup): Calories 223, Fat 23g, Carbohydrates 5g, Protein 4g

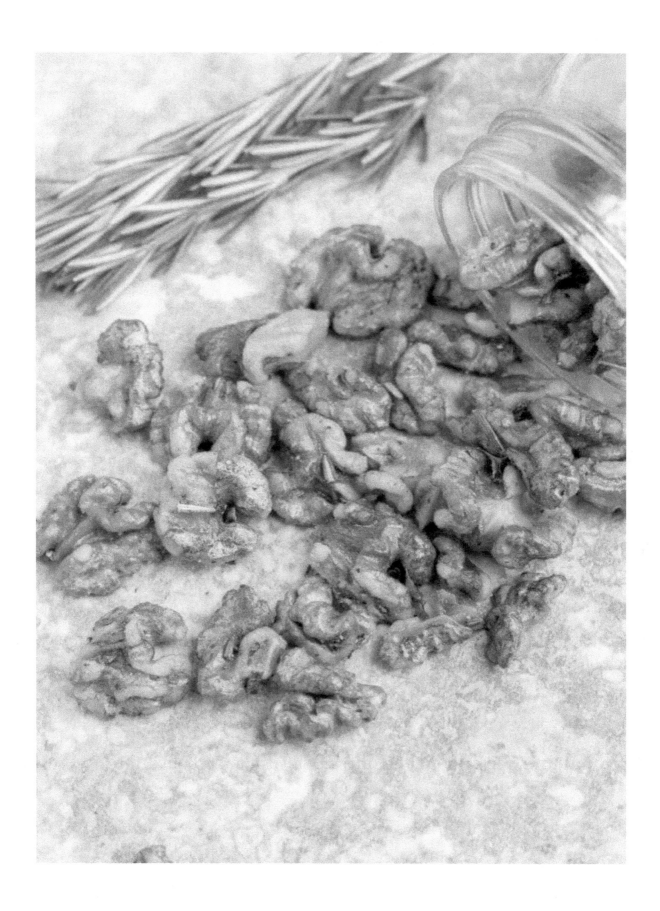

Cream Cheese Stuffed Celery

Celery sticks stuffed with cream cheese, bacon and topped with walnut chips are outrageously good!

Ingredients: 12 servings

- 10 stalks celery, rinsed and dried well
- 16 oz (2 packages) cream cheese, softened to room temperature
- 1 tablespoon milk
- 1 ¼ oz (1 packet) vegetable soup mix
- ½ cup walnut chips
- ½ cup bacon pieces, for topping

Directions:

- Cut dried celery stalks into 3 section each. Set aside.
- In a bowl, using an electric mixer, combine cream cheese and milk together. Add dry vegetable soup mix and stir well.
- Stuff celery with cream cheese mixture. If your mixture is thin enough, you can use a piping bag with tip and pipe the stuffing into the celery.
- Sprinkle with walnut chips or bacon pieces (optional). Enjoy!

Nutritional info per serving: Calories 208, Fat 18g, Carbohydrates 9g, Protein 5g

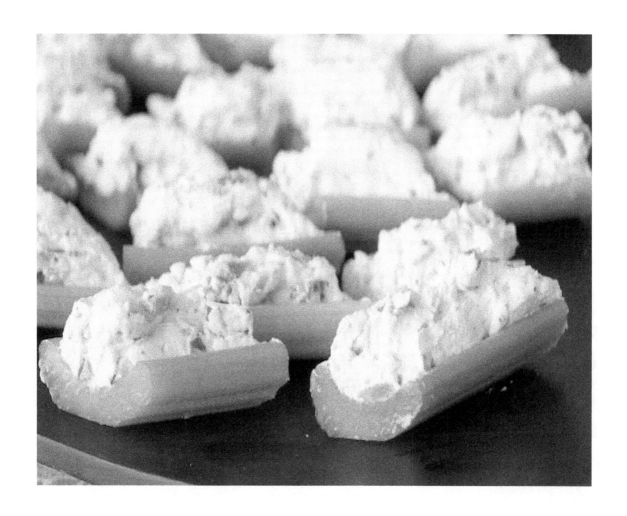

Baked Artichoke & Cilantro Pizza Dipping Sauce

Add a little sophistication to your day with this Baked Artichoke and Cilantro Pizza Dipping Sauce! Serve it with chips, nachos, bread or veggies!

Ingredients: 6 servings

- 1 – 6.5 oz jar artichoke hearts, drained and chopped
- ½ cup pizza sauce, preferably with garlic
- 2 tablespoons fresh cilantro
- ¾ cup Parmesan cheese, grated
- 1/3 cup light mayonnaise

Garnish:

- Fresh cilantro sprigs

Directions:

- Heat oven to 350° F. Mix all of the dip ingredients together and spoon into a shallow ovenproof dish or 9 inch pie plate sprayed with non-stick cooking spray.
- Bake 20 minutes until hot and bubbly.
- Garnish with cilantro sprigs and serve warm. Serve with chips, nachos, bread or veggies. Enjoy!

Nutritional info per serving: Calories 88, Fat 5g, Carbohydrates 2g, Protein 3g

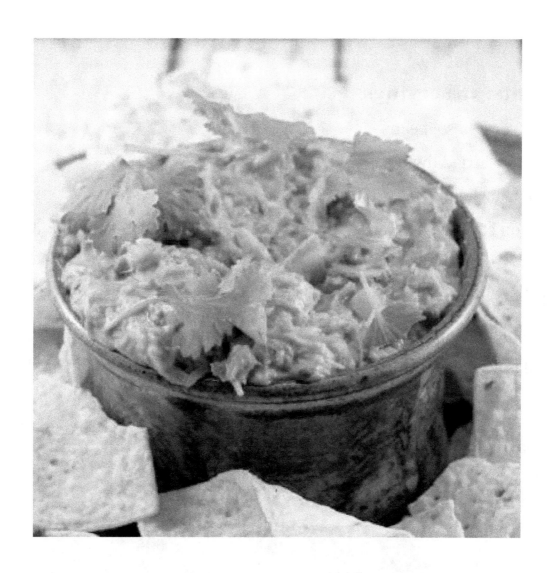

Herbed Soy Snacks

These easy soybean snacks have a great crunch and are very versatile! Give them a kick with cayenne pepper or chili powder!

Ingredients: 16 servings

- 2 cups dry roasted soybeans
- 1 ½ teaspoons dried thyme, crushed
- ¼ teaspoon garlic salt
- 1/8 teaspoon cayenne pepper

Directions:

- In a 15x10 inch baking pan spread roasted soybeans in an even layer.

- In a small bowl combine thyme, garlic salt, and cayenne pepper. Sprinkle soybeans with thyme mixture. Bake in a 350° F oven about 5 minutes or until heated through, shaking pan once. Cool completely and enjoy!

Nutritional info per serving (2 cups): Calories 75, Fat 3g, Carbohydrates 4g, Protein 7g

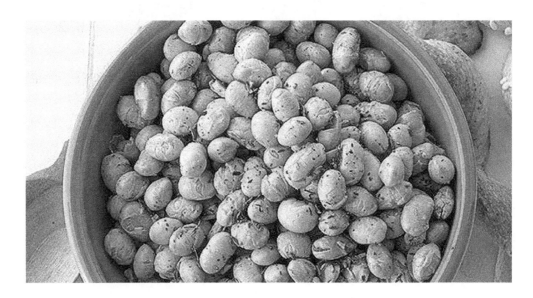

Desserts

Cinnamon & Cardamom Bombs

Small, but delicious! With familiar flavors of vanilla, cinnamon and cardamom, this is the perfect dessert!

Ingredients: 10 servings
- ¼ teaspoon ground cinnamon
- ¼ teaspoon ground cardamom
- ½ teaspoon vanilla extract
- 3 oz unsalted butter
- ½ cup unsweetened shredded coconut

Directions:
- Bring the butter to room temperature.
- Roast the shredded coconut carefully until they turn a little brown. This will create a delicious flavor, but you can skip this if you want. Let cool.
- Mix together butter, half of the shredded coconut and spices in a bowl.
- Form into walnut-sized balls with two teaspoons. Roll in the rest of the shredded coconut. Serva and enjoy!

Nutritional info per serving: Calories 90, Fat 8g, Carbohydrates 0.9g, Protein 0.7g

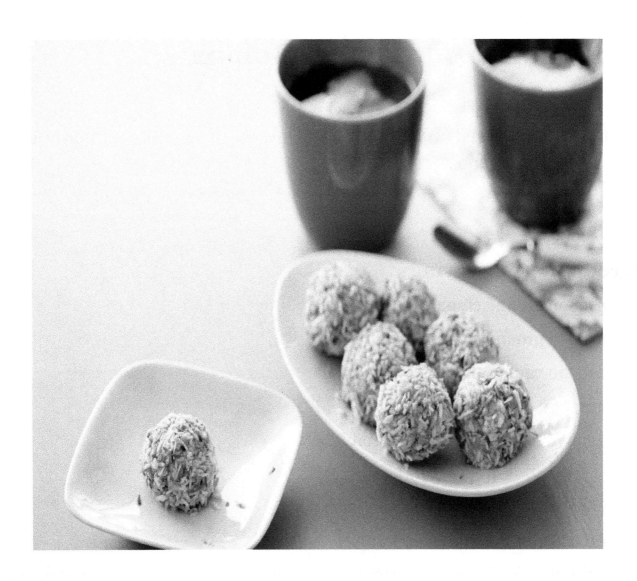

Blueberry Cupcakes

These blueberry cupcakes are baked with coconut flour and topped with a blueberry cream cheese topping. A colorful and tasty cupcake for an afternoon treat!

Ingredients: 6 cupcakes

Cupcake Mixture:
- ¼ cup butter, melted
- ¼ cup coconut flour
- ¼ cup erythritol
- 5 tablespoons blueberry blended mixture
- 3 eggs
- ½ teaspoon baking powder
- 1 teaspoon vanilla extract
- ¼ teaspoon salt

Frosting:
- ¼ cup butter, softened
- 4 oz cream cheese, softened
- 5 tablespoons blueberry blended mixture
- 1 tablespoon erythritol
- ½ teaspoon vanilla extract

Directions:

Blueberry Mixture:

• Place the blueberries in a blender and blitz. Set aside.

Cupcakes:

• Blend the butter, eggs, erythritol and vanilla essence.

• Add the coconut flour , baking powder and salt. Whisk until the batter is smooth.

• Add the blueberry mixture and combine thoroughly.

• Pour the batter into cupcake cups.

• Bake for 30 minutes until firm at 400° F.

• Remove from the oven and allow to cool.

Frosting:

• Blend the butter, cream cheese, erythritol and vanilla until smooth.

• Add the blueberry blend and mix until combined. You might want to add more blueberries for a different color.

• Pipe or slather the mixture on top of the cupcakes. Serve and enjoy!

Nutritional info per serving (1 cupcake): Calories 253, Fat 19g, Carbohydrates 4g, Protein 5g

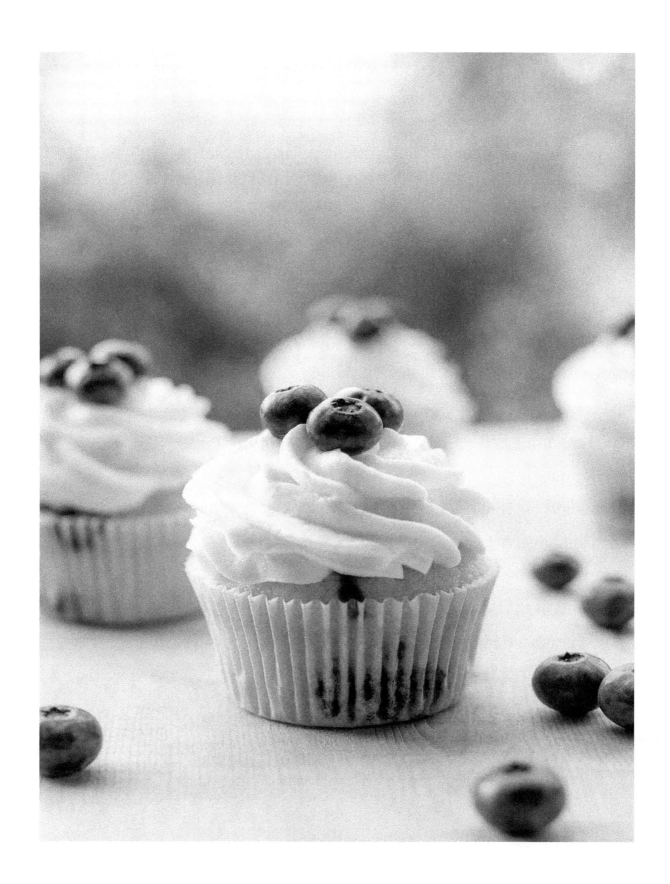

Chocolate Cake with Chocolate Glaze

This chocolate cake proves that sinful-tasting desserts don't have to make you feel foggy and fatigued! With a perfect crumb and a silky chocolate glaze, this cake is free from grains, sugar, and milk, but still delivers perfect fudgy flavor in every bite!

Ingredients: 8 servings

Chocolate Cake:

- ½ cup coconut flour
- 2 teaspoons vanilla extract, or 1 teaspoon vanilla powder
- ½ cup coconut cream
- ½ cup coconut oil, melted
- ½ cup cacao powder
- 5 eggs, separated
- 4 tablespoons granulated sweetener
- Additional grass-fed butter, ghee, or coconut oil for greasing
- Pinch of salt

Chocolate Glaze:

- 1 tablespoon ghee or coconut oil
- 1 cup coconut cream
- 1 tablespoon cacao powder
- 1 teaspoon vanilla extract
- 1 tablespoon erythritol
- Pinch of salt

Directions:

- Preheat the oven to 350° F. Grease an 8 inch metal cake pan with coconut oil.

- Whisk egg whites until they develop a foamy consistency.

- In a separate bowl, mix all remaining chocolate cake ingredients. Then slowly fold egg whites into the batter.

- Pour batter into cake pan. Bake for 25 minutes, or until a knife inserted into the center of the cake comes out clean.

- While chocolate cools, prepare glaze. In a saucepan on low heat, add all glaze ingredients and whisk continuously to combine.

- Pour chocolate glaze into a glass jar and drizzle over the cake. Serve chocolate cake warm, or store covered on your counter or in the refrigerator.

Nutritional info per serving: Calories 321, Fat 27g, Carbohydrates 4.9g, Protein 6.5g

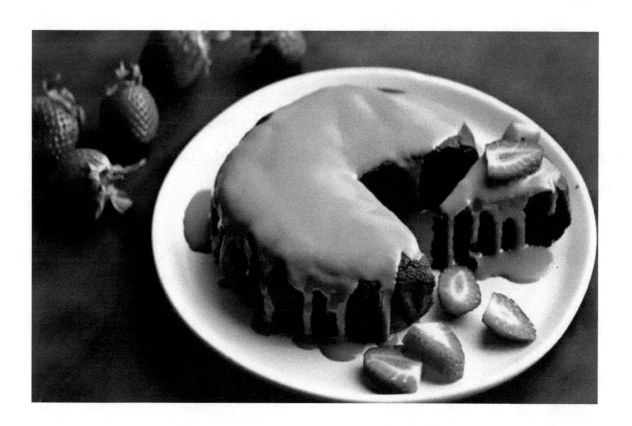

Coconut Strawberry Mousse

This coconut strawberry mousse is a lighter mousse compared to the heavier cream based ones. If your coconut cream isn't high enough in fat, then keep your tin of coconut cream in the fridge as the heavy coconut cream hardens and settles at the top, making it easy to skim off and whip.

Ingredients: 4 servings

- 1 ¾ cups coconut cream
- 1 cup strawberries, diced
- 1-2 teaspoon granulated sweetener

Directions:

- Whisk the coconut cream until fluffy and light.
- In a small bowl, add the strawberries and sweetener. Using the blade attachment on the stick blender, puree until smooth.
- Gently fold the strawberry mixture with the fluffy coconut cream.
- Serve in glasses and garnish with a few extra pieces of strawberry.
- Refrigerate or freeze as you like.

Nutritional info per serving: Calories 253, Fat 22.7g, Carbohydrates 3.9g, Protein 2.8g

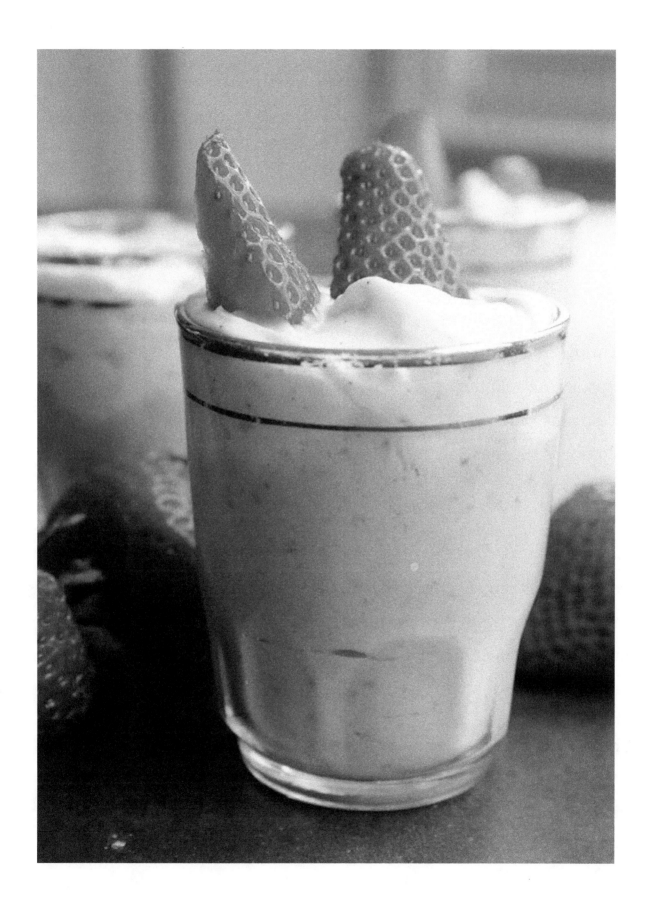

Avocado Popsicles

Avocado Popsicles are one of the best and healthiest options for those summer days. Your family will love you for giving them something yummy!

Ingredients: 6 servings

- 2 medium avocados
- 2/3 cup low-carb chocolate
- 1 cup unsweetened almond milk
- 2 teaspoons cacao butter
- 2 tablespoons lemon juice
- 6 tablespoons sugar alternative
- Chocolate ganache

Directions:

- Place 2 avocados, lemon juice, and sugar alternative into the mixer and mix properly.
- Fill all of the molds with the mixture and place it into the freezer to freeze.
- In the meantime, melt chocolate and cacao butter in a double container.
- Once the ice pops are frozen, take each one and dip it into the cooled chocolate. The chocolate can't be too hot, otherwise, it will melt the popsicle as well.
- Eat it straight or place it back into the freezer for later. Enjoy!

Nutritional info per serving: Calories 43, Fat 3g, Carbohydrates 2g, Protein 1g

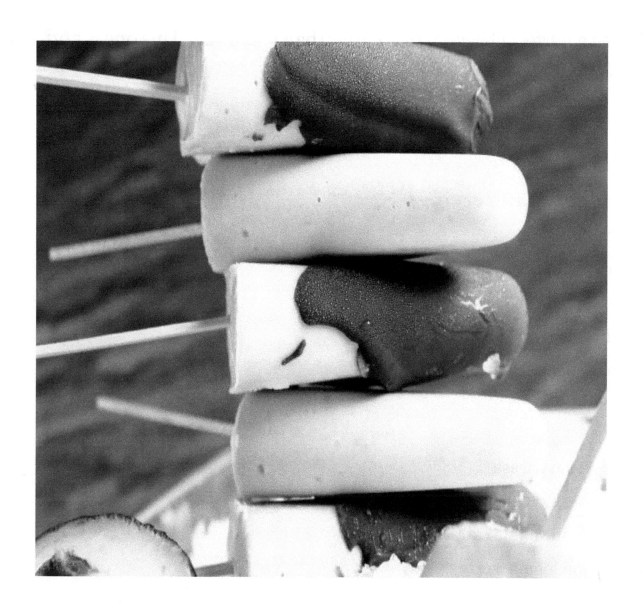

Cheesecake with Blueberries

Making a perfect cheesecake is easier than you think! This one is both sugar and gluten-free, yet still tastes like a dream! Rich and comforting creaminess, topped with juicy fresh blueberries.

Ingredients: 12 servings

Crust:
- 1 ¼ cups almond flour
- ½ teaspoon vanilla extract
- 2 oz butter
- 2 tablespoons erythritol

Filling:
- 20 oz cream cheese
- ½ cup fresh blueberries
- ½ teaspoon vanilla extract
- 1 teaspoon lemon, zest
- 2 eggs
- 1 egg yolk
- ½ cup heavy whipping cream or crème fraîche
- 1 tablespoon erythritol

Directions:

- Preheat the oven to 350° F. Butter a 9 inch springform pan and line the base with parchment paper.

- Melt the butter for the crust and heat until it gets a nutty scent. This will give the crust a lovely toffee flavor.

- Remove from heat and add almond flour, vanilla and sweetener. Combine into a dough and press into the base of the springform pan. Bake for 8 minutes, until the crust turns lightly golden. Set aside and allow to cool while you prepare the filling.

- Mix together cream cheese, heavy cream, eggs, lemon zest, vanilla and sweetener, if you're using any. Combine well. Pour the mixture over the crust.

- Raise the heat to 400° F and bake for 15 minutes.

- Lower the heat to 230° F and bake for another 45-60 minutes.

- Turn off the heat and let it cool in the oven. Remove when it has cooled completely and place it in the fridge to rest overnight. Serve with fresh blueberries.

Nutritional info per serving: Calories 315, Fat 28g, Carbohydrates 5g, Protein 7g

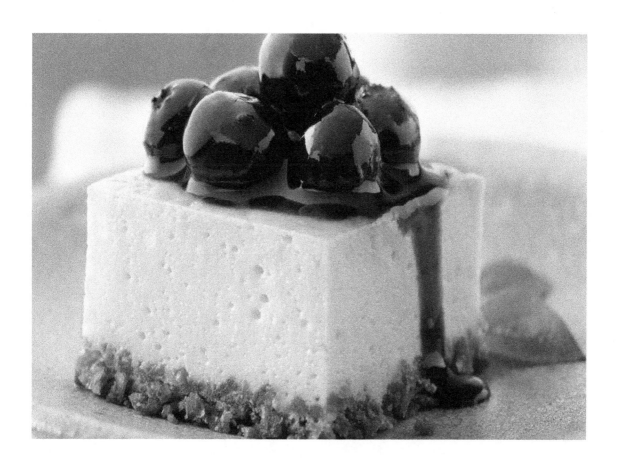

Coconut Lime Bars

These Lime Bars are a go-to easy sweet treat for warm weather, since they require no baking. Plus, they pack every light bite with powerful, healthy ingredients.

Ingredients: 10 servings

Lime Bars:
- 4 tablespoons lime juice, plus zest
- 4 cups desiccated coconut
- 3 teaspoons vanilla extract
- 4 tablespoons coconut oil
- 6 tablespoons collagen peptides
- 2 tablespoons erythritol
- Pinch of salt

Matcha Topping:
- 1 teaspoon matcha
- 1 tablespoon lime juice
- ½ cup coconut cream
- 2 tablespoons coconut oil
- 1 teaspoon vanilla extract, or ½ teaspoon vanilla powder
- ½ tablespoon liquid stevia to taste

Directions:
Lime Bars:

- In a blender, add desiccated coconut and blitz until fine, stopping to scrape down the sides of the blender as needed.

- Add all the remaining vanilla slice ingredients except collagen and blend until fine and well combined.

- Add collagen, and blend on the lowest setting until just mixed.

- Taste the mixture and add more lime juice or sweetener, if desired.

- Line a small loaf tin with parchment paper, add the mix, and press down gently with your hands or the back of a spoon until even and compact.

- Place in the freezer until firm.

Matcha Topping:

- In a saucepan on low heat, add all topping ingredients and melt together. Use a fork or whisk, or blend for a few seconds on medium speed so it combines well.

- Place the mix in a small bowl, and then into your fridge to set slightly.

- To serve, cut your lime bars into pieces and scoop the matcha mixture on top.

Nutritional info per serving: Calories 172, Fat 12.3g, Carbohydrates 2.7g, Protein 3.8g

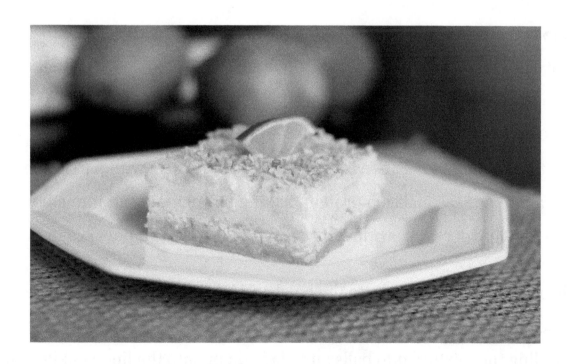

Chocolate Cookies

These protein cookies take about as much time to make as the conventional recipes you're used to while providing nutrient-dense fats and gut-healing collagen protein!

Ingredients: 16 cookies

- 2 cups organic almond meal
- 2 teaspoons vanilla
- 1 teaspoon apple cider vinegar
- 1/3 cup sugar-free chocolate, chopped
- 1 pastured egg
- ½ teaspoon baking powder
- 3 tablespoons collagen protein
- 3 tablespoons grass-fed ghee or butter
- Stevia to taste
- Pinch of salt

Directions:

- Preheat the oven to 340° F. Grease and line 2 baking trays with parchment paper.
- Add the almond meal, collagen protein, baking powder and salt into a bowl.
- Pour the apple cider vinegar directly on top of the baking powder and allow it to react.
- Add the remaining ingredients to the bowl and stir to combine evenly.
- Taste the dough and adjust the sweetness if needed.
- Begin rolling the mixture into balls and place them onto the lined baking tray.

- Press the balls as flat as you like, they won't rise much, so if you like them softer and chewier keep them quite full. However, if you like a crunchier cookie, press them quite flat using your hands to shape them.

- Place the cookies in the oven and bake for 15 minutes, or until golden brown.

- Remove from the oven when they're ready and place the cookies on a wire cooling rack.

Nutritional info per serving: Calories 118, Fat 11g, Carbohydrates 2.6g, Protein 5.5g

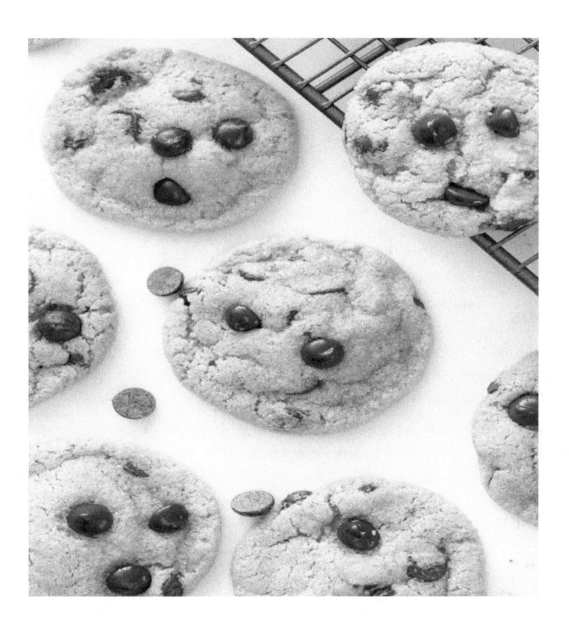

Pistachio Pudding

This Pistachio Pudding is unbelievably delicious! Enjoy it!

Ingredients: 6 servings

- 1 cup raw unsalted pistachios, shelled, plus more for garnish
- 2 cups plus 2 tablespoons whole milk, divided
- 1 large egg plus 2 parge egg yolks
- ¼ tablespoon pure vanilla extract
- ½ cup granulated sugar, divided
- 2 tablespoons unsalted butter
- 2 tablespoons cornstarch
- 1/8 teaspoon salt
- Whipped cream, for garnish

Directions:

- Add pistachios to the bowl of a food processor and process until finely ground and beginning to thicken, about 3-4 minutes. Add ¼ cup sugar and 2 tablespoons milk and pulse until a paste forms.

- Combine the paste with the remaining 2 cups milk in a large saucepan and cook over medium-high heat, whisking to break up any clumps, until the mixture begins to steam. While the milk is heating, add the remaining ¼ cup sugar with the egg, yolks, cornstarch, and salt to the food processor and process until combined. With the food processor still running, slowly add ½ cup of the warm milk into the mixture to temper the eggs.

- Scrape the contents of the food processor into the saucepan with the remaining warm milk mixture and cook over medium heat, stirring constantly, until the pudding starts to bubble and thicken. Remove from the heat, add the butter and vanilla, and stir until the butter is melted.

• Divide the pudding among 6 servings cups. Cover each with plastic wrap pressed directly against the surface of the puddings. Chill for at least 4 hours.

• Serve topped with whipped cream and chopped pistachios.

Nutritional info per serving: Calories 301, Fat 16g, Carbohydrates 26g, Protein 10g

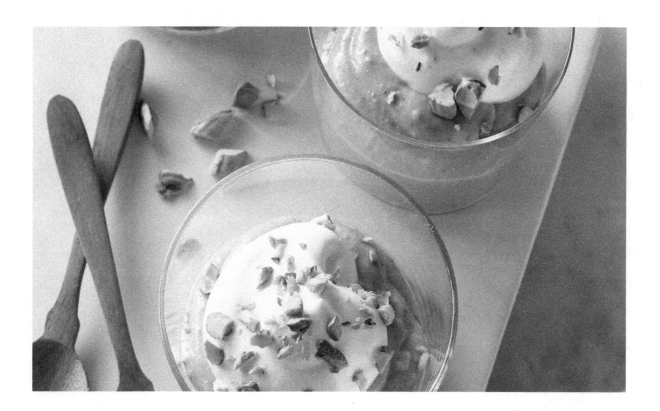

Apple Berry Crumble Pies

Use tayberry for this pie, which are a raspberry/blackberry hybrid! They taste so good!

Ingredients: 2 servings

- 2 medium firm apples, peeled and cut into ¼ inch slices
- 1 pie crust
- 1 ½ cups frozen berries (tayberries, raspberries, and blueberries)
- 4 teaspoons tapioca flour
- 1 teaspoon cinnamon
- 1/3 cup light brown sugar
- 1/3 cup white sugar
- ¼ teaspoon salt

Crumble Topping:

- ½ cup rolled oats
- 1/3 cup walnuts, chopped
- ½ cup all-purpose flour
- 6 tablespoons unsalted butter, cold and cut into cubes
- ¼ cup granulated sugar
- ¼ cup light brown sugar

Directions:

- Preheat oven to 375° F. Line two 4 inch ceramic ramekins with rolled out pie crust. Press crust into ramekins and repair any tears with extra pie crust. Place in freezer until ready to fill pie.

- For Filling: Use a medium saucepan to combine apples and brown sugar. Cook over medium-low heat for about 10 minutes, until reduced and bubbling.

- Drain most juice from apples, and add berries, tapioca flour, sugar, cinnamon, and salt and stir gently to combine.

- For crumble: Mix together all ingredients except butter. Add butter and cut into mixture with pastry cutter or fork until it resembles coarse crumbs.

- Remove pie crust from freezer and add apple-berry filling until ramekin is full. Add generous handful of crumble topping by packing it on.

- Bake for 25 minutes; the top of the pie should be starting to turn golden brown. Tent with foil and bake for another 10 to 15 minutes until filling is bubbling.

- Remove from oven and let cool for 15 minutes. Serve warm and enjoy!

Nutritional info per serving: Calories 214, Fat 7.9g, Carbohydrates 28g, Protein 2.7g

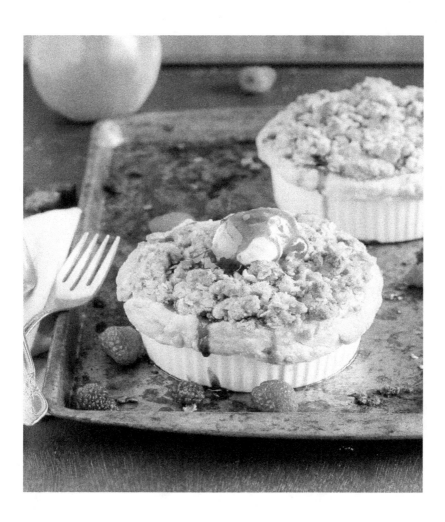

Mocha Truffle Cheesecake

This cheesecake is ideal for get-togethers because it can be made in advance! Its brownie-like crust and creamy mocha layer really hit the spot!

Ingredients: 16 servings

- 1 to 3 tablespoons instant coffee granules
- 1 package devil's food cake mix, regular size
- 1 large egg, room temperature
- 6 tablespoons butter, melted

Filling/Topping:

- 2 packages (8 oz each) cream cheese, softened
- 1 can sweetened condensed milk
- 3 to 6 tablespoons instant coffee granules
- 3 large eggs, room temperature, lightly beaten
- 2 cups semisweet chocolate chips, melted and cooled
- 1 cup heavy whipping cream
- ½ teaspoon almond extract
- 1 tablespoon baking cocoa
- ¼ cup confectioners' sugar
- ¼ cup hot water

Directions:

- In a large bowl, combine the cake mix, butter, egg, and coffee granules until well blended. Press onto the bottom and 2 inch up the sides of a greased 10 inch springform pan.

- In another large bowl, beat cream cheese until smooth. Beat in milk and melted chips. Dissolve coffee granulates in water. Add to cream cheese mixture. Add eggs. Beat on low speed just until combined. Pour into crust. Place pan on a baking sheet.

- Bake at 325° F until center is almost set, about 50-55 minutes. Cool on a wire rack for 10 minutes. Carefully run a knife around edge of pan to loosen. Cool 1 hour longer. Chill overnight.

- Just before serving, in a large bowl, beat cream until soft peaks form. Beat in sugar and extract until stiff peaks form. Spread over top of cheesecake. Sprinkle with cocoa if desired. Refrigerate leftovers.

Nutritional info per serving (1 slice): Calories 424, Fat 22g, Carbohydrates 48g, Protein 8g

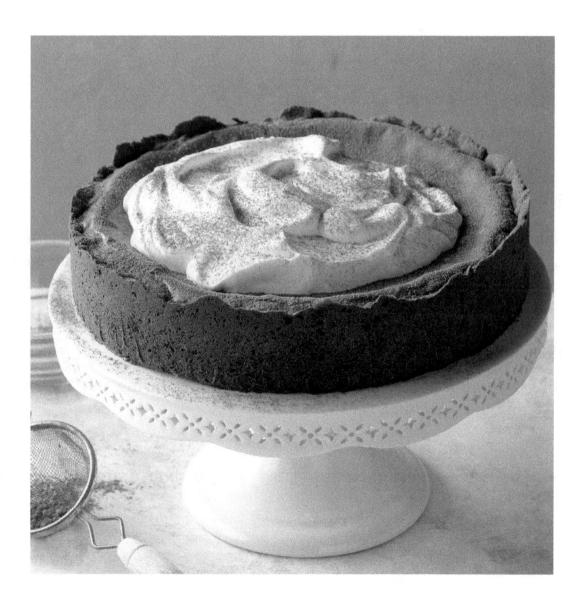

Vanilla Cheesecake Popsicles

These Vanilla Cheesecake Pops taste so rich and utterly sinful, but they're just 128 calories each!

Ingredients: 8 popsicles

- 1 vanilla bean, seeds scraped
- 8 oz light cream cheese
- 1 teaspoon vanilla extract
- ½ cup low-fat milk
- ½ cup non-fat plain or vanilla Greek yogurt
- 2/3 cup powdered sugar

Directions:

- Place all ingredients into a food processor. To scrape the seeds from the vanilla bean, cut through one layer vertically with a paring knife and then, using the back of the paring knife, scrape down the inside of the bean to remove the seeds. Add seeds to mixture and discard the rest of the bean. Pulse until ingredients are completely blended. Divide mixture between 8 popsicle molds and add sticks. Freeze for 3-4 hours until solid.

- To remove from molds, hold mold upside down under warm water and gently tug on the stick until the pop comes out.

Nutritional info per serving: Calories 118, Fat 6g, Carbohydrates 10g, Protein 1.8g

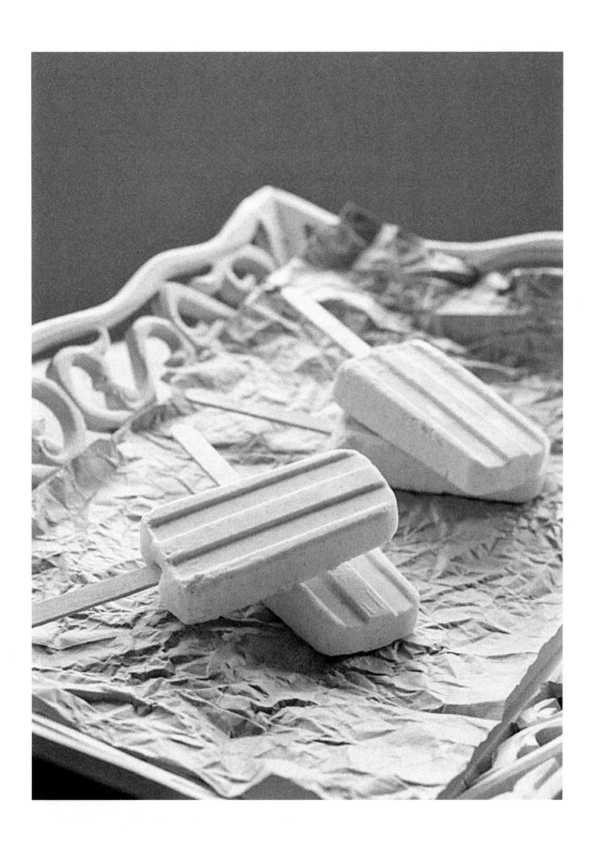

Balsamic Plum Ice Cream

This Balsamic Plum Ice Cream is better than whatever you were going to buy at the grocery store!

Ingredients: 3-4 cups

- 9 medium-small plums, halved and destoned
- ¼ cup balsamic vinegar
- 1 tablespoon tapioca powder
- ½ cup maple syrup

Ice Cream Mixture:

- 1 cup raw cashews, pre-soaked and strained
- 1 teaspoon pure vanilla extract
- 1 cup unsweetened dairy-free yogurt
- ½ cup maple syrup
- 1/8 teaspoon ground cardamom
- ¼ teaspoon salt

Directions:

- Combine all plum mixture ingredients in a medium-small saucepan and bring to a light boil on medium-high heat. Once the mixture begins to bubble, continue simmering for 10 minutes, stirring occasionally. Remove from heat and cool on a wire rack until mixture is at room temperature.

- Blend all ice cream mixture ingredients as well as the cooled plum mixture in a high power blender until smooth.

- Transfer into a freezer-safe container and chill for 5-6 hours or overnight. Thaw out on the counter before serving and enjoy!

Nutritional info per serving: Calories 149, Fat 7g, Carbohydrates 12.8g, Protein 1.3g

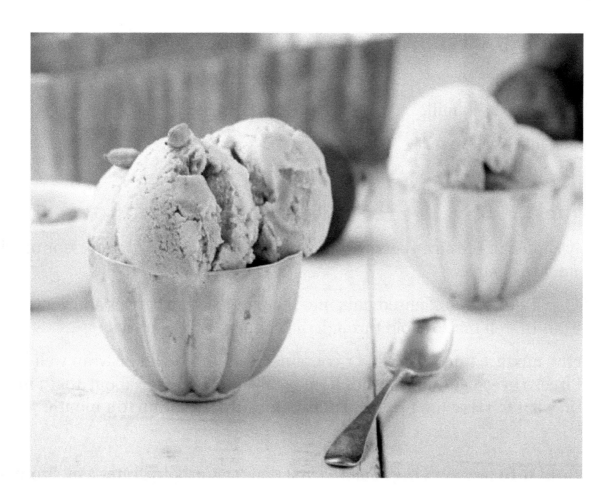

Frozen Strawberry Yogurt

This gorgeous Frozen Strawberry Yogurt is intensely fruity and really creamy!

Ingredients: 5 servings

- ¾ cup strawberries
- 1 cup light condensed milk
- 2 cups 0%-fat Greek yogurt

Directions:

• Roughly chop half the strawberries and whizz the rest in a food processor or with a stick blender to a purèe.

• In a big bowl, stir the condensed milk into the purèed strawberries and gently stir in the yogurt until well mixed. Fold through the chopped strawberries.

• Scrape the mixture into a loaf tin or container, pop on the lid or wrap well in cling film and freeze overnight, until solid. Remove from the freezer about 10-15 minutes before you want to serve the frozen yogurt. Can be frozen for up to 1 month.

Nutritional info per serving: Calories 164, Fat 0g, Carbohydrates 27g, Protein 12g

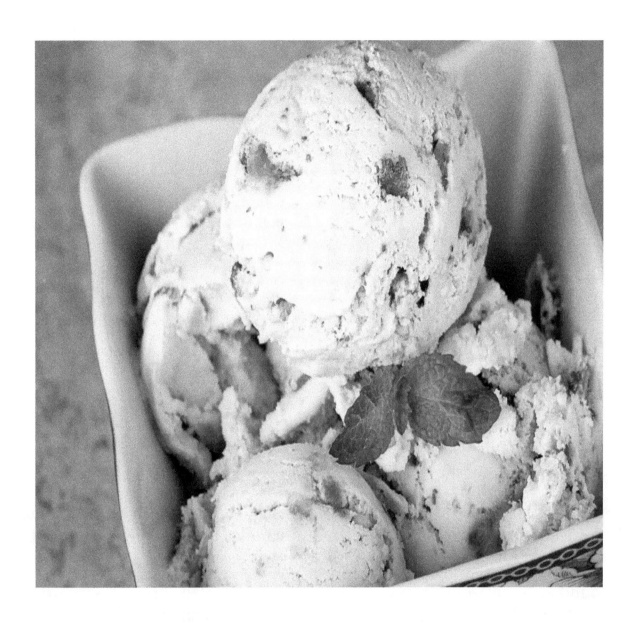

Raspberry-Lemon Cream Cake

This Raspberry-Lemon Cream Cake is going to win over anyone!

Ingredients: 12 servings

- 2 cups raspberries
- ½ cup prepared lemon curd
- ¼ teaspoon vanilla extract
- 3 tablespoons red raspberry jam
- 2 oz cream cheese
- 3 tablespoons confectioners' sugar
- 1 cup whipping cream
- 1 frozen all-butter pound cake

Directions:

- To prepare frosting, beat cream cheese and sugar in a large bowl, with mixer at medium speed, until smooth. Add cream and vanilla. Beat on high speed until stiff peaks form. Refrigerate frosting while assembling the cake.

- Cut pound cake horizontally into 3 equal-size slices. Place bottom slice on platter and spread with ¼ cup lemon curd. Arrange ¾ cup raspberries over lemon curd. Spread jam on one side of each of the two remaining slices of pound cake. Repeat process with remaining ¼ cup lemon curd, ¾ cup raspberries and remaining cake. Spread frosting over top and sides of cake, cover loosely with plastic wrap and refrigerate 2 hours or overnight.

- Garnish cake with lemon peel and remaining ½ cup raspberries. Cut into slices with a serrated knife.

Nutritional info per serving: Calories 348, Fat 16g, Carbohydrates 43g, Protein 7g

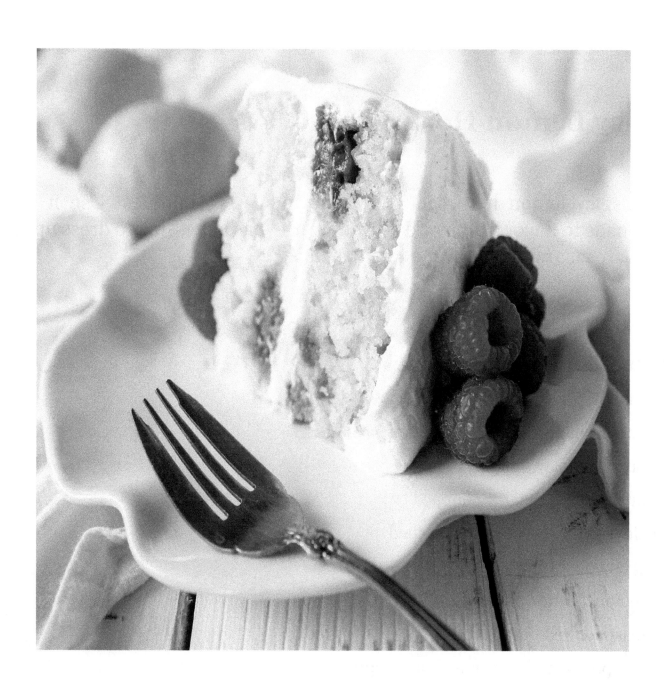

Dressings

Spicy Lemon Herb Sauce

This spicy lemon herb sauce is ready in just 15 minutes! Use it as a marinade to flavor dish, pork or tofu. Or use it as a dressing to dress up any salad, from grains to chicken to greens.

Ingredients: 2 servings
- 1 shallot, peeled and roughly chopped
- 1 bunch cilantro, roughly chopped
- 1 bunch parsley, roughly chopped
- 1 bunch mint, roughly chopped
- 1 clove garlic, peeled and smashed
- 1/3 cup olive oil
- 2 lemons, zested and juiced
- 1 teaspoon red pepper flakes
- 2 teaspoons freshly ground black pepper
- 1 teaspoon salt

Directions:
- In a blender or food processor, pulse the shallot, garlic, herbs, and lemon zest to combine.

• Add the lemon juice and olive oil, then pulse until a smooth sauce forms. Season with salt, pepper and red pepper flakes.

• Transfer the sauce to an airtight container and refrigerate until ready to use. The sauce will keep for up to a week.

Nutritional info per serving: Calories 370, Fat 31g, Carbohydrates 8g, Protein 6g

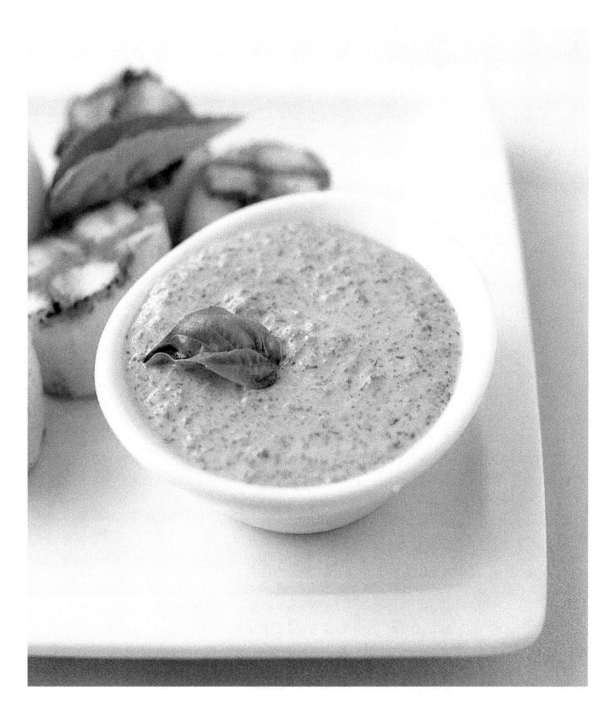

Shallots & Red Wine Sauce

This classic French sauce is just perfect with a rib-eye steak!

Ingredients: 4 servings

- 2 cups shallots, sliced
- 14 fl oz red wine
- 14 fl oz beef stock or brown chicken stock
- 1 garlic clove, lightly crushed
- 4 tablespoons olive oil
- 5 tablespoons balsamic vinegar
- Spring rosemary
- Knob of butter
- Salt, to taste
- Ground black pepper, to season

Directions:

- Sautè 2 cups sliced shallots in a medium saucepan with 4 tablespoons olive oil over a high heat for about 3 minutes until lightly browned, stirring often.

- Season with ground black pepper and add 1 lightly crushed garlic clove and a sprig of rosemary.

- Continue cooking for a further 3 minutes, stirring often to prevent the shallots burning.

- Pour in 5 tablespoons balsamic vinegar and cook until evaporated away to a syrup, then pour in 14 fl oz red wine and cook until reduced by two-thirds.

- Pour in 14 fl oz beef or brown chicken stock and bring to a boil.

- Turn down the heat and simmer until reduced by two-thirds again. Remove the garlic and rosemary.
- Add a little salt to taste and whisk in a knob of butter. Add any juices from the steaks just before serving.

Nutritional info per serving: Calories 59, Fat 2.2g, Carbohydrates 2.9g, Protein 1.3g

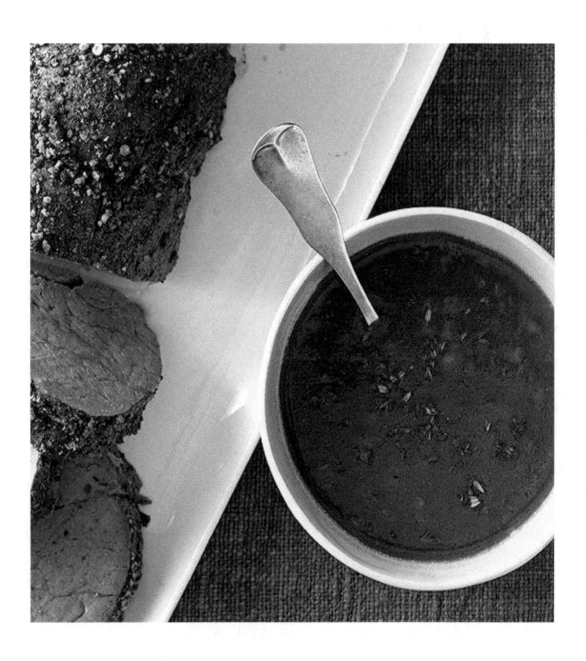

Italian Mayonnaise

Simple, pure ingredients combine in this creamy condiment that delivers zest for days. The perfect complement for salads, omelets, and Italian cold cuts such as mortadella, prosciutto and pancetta.

Ingredients: 4 servings

- 1 cup mayonnaise
- 1 tablespoon Italian seasoning

Italian Seasoning:

- 3 tablespoons dried oregano
- 3 tablespoons dried parsley
- 3 tablespoons dried basil
- 1 tablespoon garlic powder
- 1 teaspoon dried thyme
- 1 teaspoon dried rosemary
- 1 teaspoon onion powder
- 1 teaspoon dried sage
- ¼ teaspoon chili flakes
- ¼ teaspoon ground black pepper
- 1 tablespoon sea salt

Directions:

- Mix mayonnaise and Italian seasoning in a small bowl.
- Set aside for 30 minutes or more to let the flavors develop. Check if it needs additional seasoning.

• Keep refrigerated for up to 4-5 days.

Italian Seasoning:

• Thoroughly mix together the spices. Pour into a jar with a tight-fitting lid.

• If you use whole seeds, grind in a grinder either in advance or when cooking.

• Keep the spices in a dark, dry and room temperature area. Small tin cans are great.

• Make a big batch to last for 4-6 months. After this the spices will lose some flavor and color. They won't go bad but will be less powerful.

Nutritional info per serving: Calories 364, Fat 39g, Carbohydrates 2g, Protein 1g

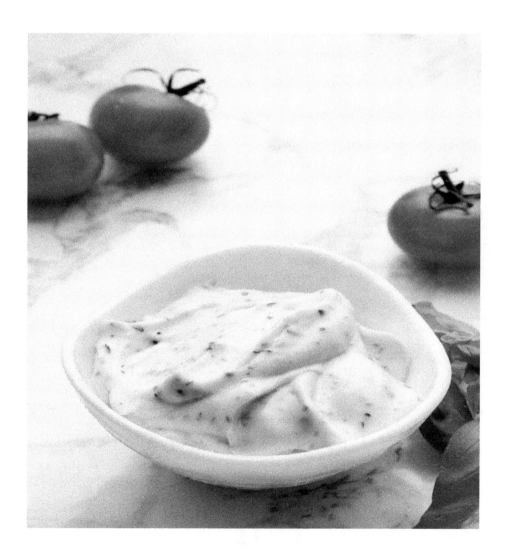

Thai Peanut Sauce

This easy peanut sauce has an amazing authentic Thai taste! It's spicy and peanutty, and is perfect as a dipping sauce for chicken, shrimp, and beef.

Ingredients: 16 servings

- 1 ½ cups creamy peanut butter
- 3 cloves garlic, minced
- ½ cup coconut milk
- 3 tablespoons fresh lime juice
- 3 tablespoons soy sauce
- ¼ cup fresh cilantro, chopped
- 1 tablespoon fresh ginger root, minced
- 1 tablespoon hot sauce
- 3 tablespoons water
- 1 tablespoon fish sauce

Directions:

- In a bowl, mix the peanut butter, coconut milk, water, lime juice, soy sauce, fish sauce, hot sauce, ginger and garlic. Mix in the cilantro just before serving.

Nutritional info per serving: Calories 160, Fat 13.7g, Carbohydrates 5.7g, Protein 6.5g

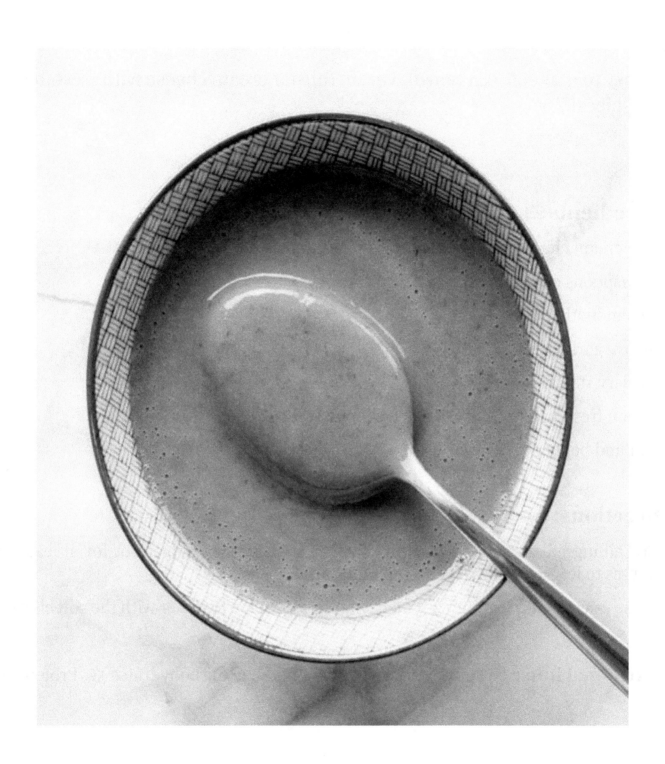

Cream Cheese with Herbs

So easy to make! Mix a non-flavored, full-fat cream cheese with fresh herbs and spices!

Ingredients: 4 servings

- 8 oz cream cheese
- 2 teaspoons olive oil
- ½ lemon, the zest
- 1 clove garlic
- 4 celery stalks
- ½ cup fresh parsley or fresh basil, chopped
- Salt and pepper to taste

Directions:

- Stir all ingredients into the cream cheese. Let sit in the refrigerator for at least 10 minutes to let all the flavors develop. Add salt if needed.

- Rinse celery stalks, cut into 2-3 inch lengths, and serve together with the soft cheese.

Nutritional info per serving: Calories 229, Fat 22g, Carbohydrates 5g, Protein 4g

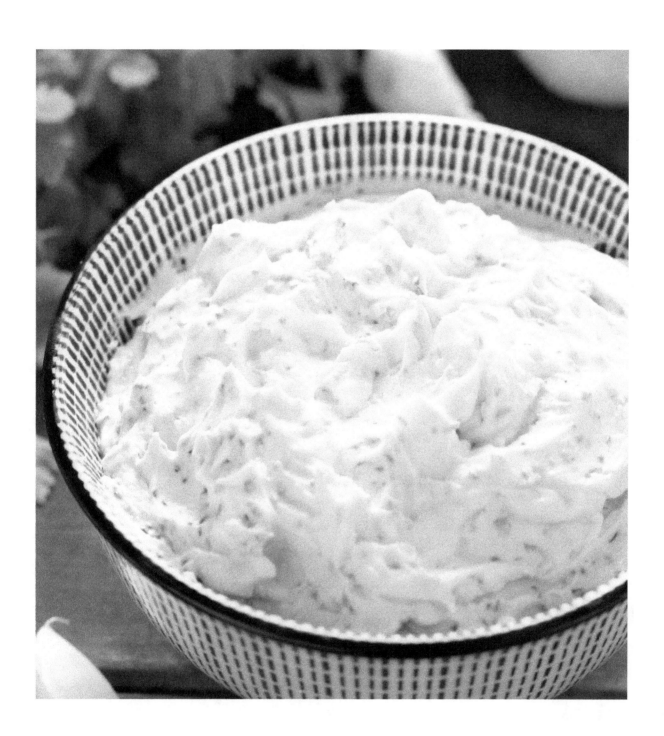

Avocado Caesar Dressing

Looking for a healthy caesar salad dressing? This Avocado Caesar Dressing uses avocado instead of eggs so it's still super creamy and flavorful, but low in calories!

Ingredients: 3-4 servings

- 1/3 cup avocado, mashed
- 2 cloves garlic, minced
- 1 tablespoon olive oil
- 2 anchovy fillets or 1 teaspoon anchovy paste
- 3 tablespoons lemon juice
- ¼ cup Parmesan cheese, shredded or shaved
- 2 tablespoons unsweetened almond milk
- 2 teaspoons Worcestershire sauce
- ½ teaspoon mustard
- 2 tablespoons water
- ¾ teaspoon sea salt
- ¼ teaspoon ground pepper

Directions:

- Add all ingredients into a high powered blender or food processor and blend until smooth. Taste and add additional salt and pepper if needed.

Nutritional info per serving (2 tablespoons): Calories 58, Fat 5g, Carbohydrates 2g, Protein 2g

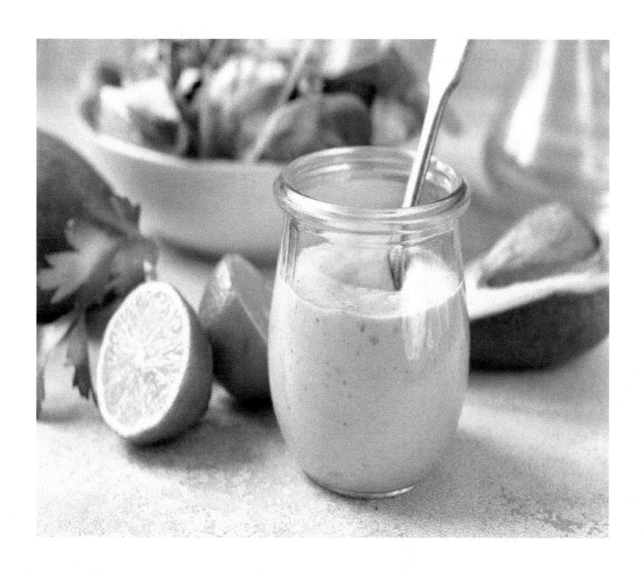

Mild Curry Seasoning

Want an exotic blend of spices without too much kick? Curry doesn't have to be hot and spicy. This flavorful blend adds flair and complexity to veggies, meat, poultry and fish.

Ingredients: 4 servings

- 2 tablespoons ground coriander seeds
- 2 tablespoons ground cumin
- ½ tablespoon yellow mustard seeds
- 2 tablespoons turmeric
- ½ tablespoon ground ginger
- ½ tablespoon chili flakes
- 1 tablespoon sea salt

Directions:

- Mix together all the spices thoroughly and pour into a jar with a tight-fitting lid.
- If you use whole seeds, grind in a grinder either in advance or just before cooking.
- Keep the spices in a dark, dry, cool place. Small tin cans are great.
- Make a batch big enough to last for about 4-6 months. After that, the spices will lose some flavor and color. They won't spoil, though, they will just be less powerful.

Nutritional info per serving: Calories 53, Fat 2g, Carbohydrates 4g, Protein 2g

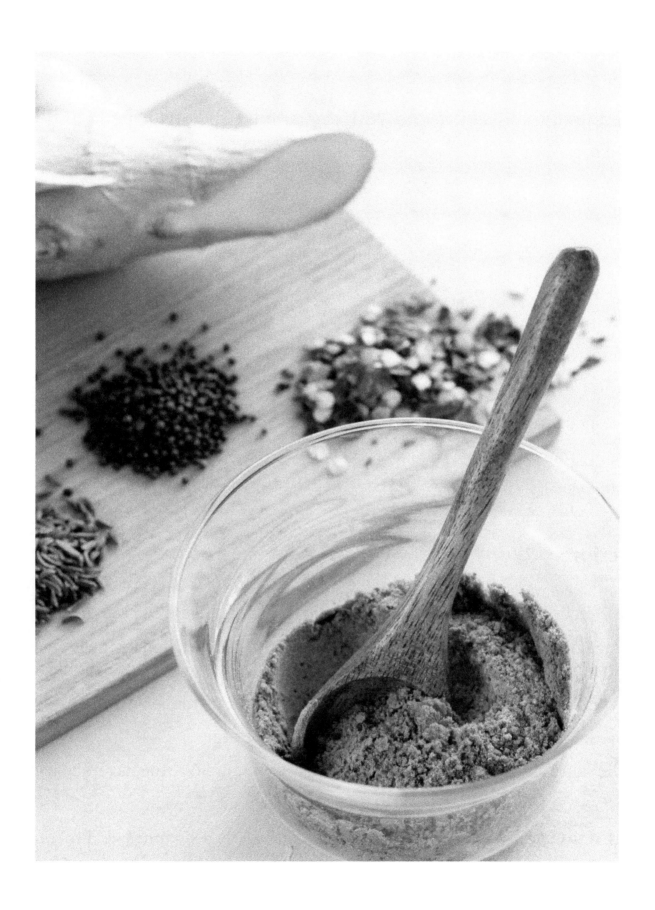

Tzatziki

Dreaming of the Greek islands? Mix up some delicious tzatziki and you'll be there!

Ingredients: 6 servings

- ½ cucumber
- 1 cup Greek yogurt
- 1 tablespoon olive oil
- 2 cloves garlic
- 1 tablespoon fresh mint, finely chopped
- Pinch of ground black pepper
- 1 teaspoon salt

Directions:

- Rinse the cucumber and chop finely. You can also grate it with the coarse side of a grater. Don't peel the cucumber. The skin adds color and texture to the sauce.

- Put cucumber in a strainer and sprinkle salt on top. Mix well and let the liquid drain for 5-10 minutes. Wrap cucumber in a tea towel and squeeze out excess liquid.

- Press or finely chop the garlic and place in a bowl. Add cucumber, oil and fresh mint.

- Stir in the yogurt and add black pepper and salt to taste.

- Let the sauce sit in the refrigerator for at least 10 minutes for the flavors to develop.

Nutritional info per serving: Calories 81, Fat 7g, Carbohydrates 3g, Protein 1g

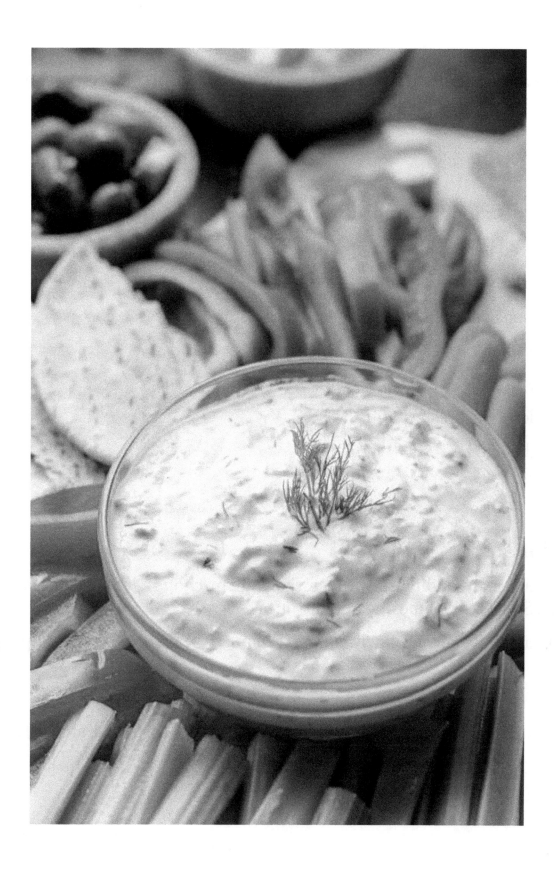

Guacamole

A little guacamole just makes life better! This foolproof recipe is perfect for a snack with veggies or on top of grilled chicken or burgers.

Ingredients: 4 servings

- 2 ripe avocados
- 1 clove garlic
- 3 tablespoons olive oil
- ½ white onion
- 1 tomato, diced
- 5 1/3 tablespoons fresh cilantro
- ½ lime, the juice
- Salt and pepper

Directions:

- Peel the avocados and mash with a fork. Grate or chop the onion finely and add to the mash. Squeeze the lime and add the juice.

- Add tomato, olive oil and finely chopped cilantro. Season with salt and pepper and mix well.

Nutritional info per serving: Calories 244, Fat 25g, Carbohydrates 5g, Protein 3g

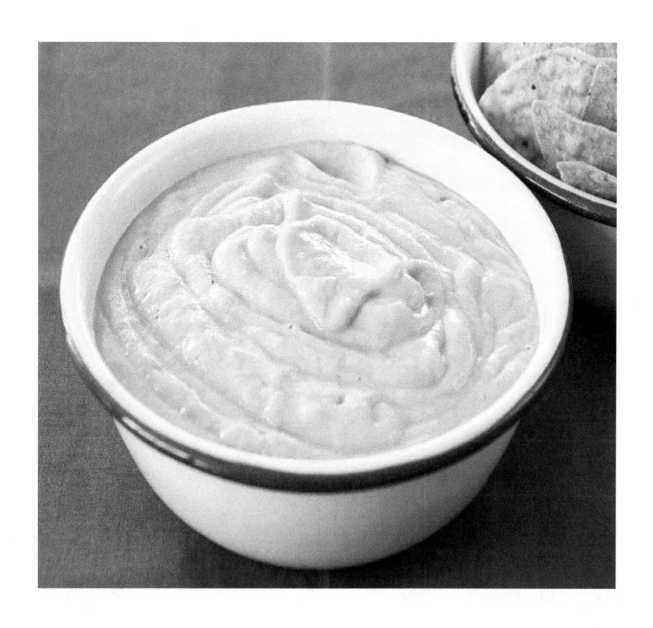

Salsa Verde

Spice up almost anything with color and a punch of flavor! Whip up a batch of salsa verde and experience enhanced pork, poultry, and fish. It also gives a huge boost to salads, cooked veggies, and egg dishes, too!

Ingredients: 4 servings

- ½ cup fresh parsley, finely chopped
- 3 tablespoons fresh basil or fresh cilantro, finely chopped
- 2 cloves garlic, crushed
- ¾ cup olive oil
- 2 tablespoons small capers
- ½ lemon, the juice
- ½ teaspoon ground black pepper
- 1 teaspoon sea salt

Directions:

- Add all of the ingredients to a deep bowl and mix with an immersion blender until the sauce has the desired consistency.
- Store the sauce in the refrigerator for up to 4-5 days or in the freezer.

Nutritional info per serving: Calories 323, Fat 37g, Carbohydrates 2g, Protein 1g

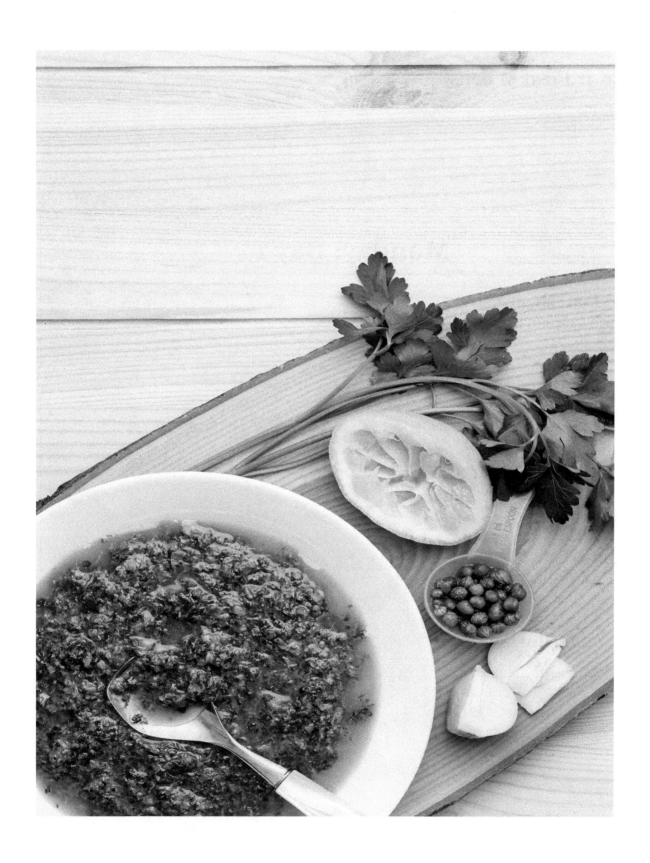

21-Day Meal Plan

Phase 1: First Week

Monday: Day 1

Breakfast: about 7.30 am
1 Sirtfood Green Juice

Mid-Morning: about 11 am
1 Sirtfood Green Juice

Snack: about 2.30 pm
1 Sirtfood Green Juice

Dinner: about 6 pm
Fish Taco Cabbage Bowl

Tot: 1022 calories

Tuesday: Day 2

Breakfast: about 7.30 am
1 Berry Turmeric Smoothie

Mid-Morning: about 11 am
1 Berry Turmeric Smoothie

Snack: about 2.30 pm
1 Berry Turmeric Smoothie

Dinner: about 6 pm
Buckwheat and Asparagus Risotto

Snack: 1 square dark chocolate (85% cocoa)

Tot: 1009 calories

Wednesday: Day 3

Breakfast: about 7.30 am
1 Mango Green Smoothie

Mid-Morning: about 11 am
1 Mango Green Smoothie

Snack: about 2.30 pm
1 Mango Green Smoothie

Dinner: about 6 pm
Avocado Tuna Salad

Snack: about 9 pm
1 square dark chocolate (85% cocoa)

Tot: 1029 calories

Thursday: Day 4

Breakfast: about 7.30 am
1 Strawberry Spinach Smoothie

Mid-Morning: about 11 am
Creamy Coconut Porridge

Snack: about 2.30 pm
1 Strawberry Spinach Smoothie

Dinner: about 6 pm
Ground Beef and Broccoli

Snack: about 9 pm
1 square dark chocolate (85% cocoa)

Tot: 1523 calories

Friday: Day 5

Breakfast: about 7.30 am
1 Carrot Celery Orange & Ginger Smoothie

Mid-Morning: about 11 am
Celery Caesar Salad

Snack: about 2.30 pm
1 Carrot Celery Orange & Ginger Smoothie

Dinner: about 6 pm
Salmon Curry

Snack: about 9 pm
1 square dark chocolate (85% cocoa)

Tot: 1494 calories

Saturday: Day 6

Breakfast: about 7.30 am
1 Blueberry Banana Avocado Smoothie

Mid-Morning: about 11 am
Coconut Yogurt Waffles

Snack: about 2.30 pm
1 Blueberry Banana Avocado Smoothie

Dinner: about 6 pm
Asian Chicken Thighs + Garlic Mushrooms

Tot: 1529 calories

Sunday: Day 7

Breakfast: about 8 am
1 Carrot Smoothie

Mid-Morning: about 10 am
1 Matcha Berry Smoothie

Lunch: about 12.30 pm
Crispy Chicken with Sweet Chili Rice

Dinner: about 6 pm
Garlic & Rosemary Grilled Lamb Chops + Cheesy Asparagus

Snack: about 9 pm
2 squares dark chocolate (85% cocoa)

Tot: 1501 calories

Phase 2: Day 8-21

Day 8 and 15

- 1 x Sirtfood green juice
- 3 x main meals
- 1 to 2 light bites or appetizers and snacks
- 1 x glass red wine

Smoothie: Ginger Plum Smoothie

Meal 1: Fresh Herbs & Cheese Scramble

Meal 2: Broccoli Salad

Meal 3: Asian Chicken Thighs

Light Bites: Tahini-Date Salted Caramels

Appetizers & Snacks: Crab Salad Stuffed Avocado

Day 9 and 16

- 1 x Sirtfood green juice
- 3 x main meals
- 1 to 2 light bites or appetizers and snacks

Smoothie: Simple Grape Smoothie

Meal 1: Sirtfood Breakfast Scramble

Meal 2: Sirtfood Salmon Salad

Meal 3: Chicken Chili

Light Bites: Buckwheat Stir Fry with Kale, Peppers & Artichokes

Appetizers & Snacks: Avocado Deviled Eggs

Day 10 and 17

- 1 x Sirtfood green juice
- 3 x main meals
- 1 to 2 light bites or appetizers and snacks
- 1 x glass red wine

Smoothie: Creamy Pineapple Cucumber Smoothie

Meal 1: Cinnamon Buckwheat Bowls

Meal 2: Kale Salad with Pecorino and Lemon

Meal 3: Macaroni & Cheese with Broccoli

Light Bites: Mixed Olive Crostini

Appetizers & Snacks: Spicy Roasted Nuts

Day 11 and 18

- 1 x Sirtfood green juice
- 3 x main meals
- 1 to 2 light bites or appetizers and snacks
- 1 to 2 squares dark chocolate (85% cocoa)

Smoothie: Tropical Watercress Juice

Meal 1: Sirtfood Omelette

Meal 2: Chia, Quinoa & Avocado Salad

Meal 3: Foil Baked Salmon

Light Bites: Walnut and Onion Tartine

Appetizers & Snacks: Broccoli Cheddar Bites

Day 12 and 19

- 1 x Sirtfood green juice
- 3 x main meals
- 1 to 2 light bites or appetizers and snacks
- 1 x glass red wine

Smoothie: Sirtfood Chocolate Strawberry Milk

Meal 1: Dark Chocolate Almond Bars

Meal 2: Herby Pork with Apple & Chicory Salad

Meal 3: Garlic Butter Roast Turkey

Light Bites: Fresh Herb Frittata

Appetizers & Snacks: Herbed Soy Snacks

Day 13 and 20

- 1 x Sirtfood green juice
- 3 x main meals
- 1 to 2 light bites or appetizers and snacks
- 1 to 2 squares dark chocolate (85% cocoa)

Smoothie: Arugula Apple Smoothie

Meal 1: Cranberry & Orange Granola

Meal 2: Arugula, Egg, and Charred Asparagus Salad

Meal 3: Fried Sardines with Olives

Light Bites: Herb-Roasted Olives and Tomatoes

Desserts: Frozen Strawberry Yogurt

Day 14 and 21

- 1 x Sirtfood green juice
- 3 x main meals
- 1 to 2 light bites or appetizers and snacks
- 1 x glass red wine

Smoothie: Sirtfood Wonder Smoothie

Meal 1: Date and Walnut Porridge

Meal 2: Grilled Asparagus with Caper Vinaigrette

Meal 3: Roast Quail with Rosemary, Thyme and Garlic

Appetizers & Snacks: Spicy Deviled Eggs

Desserts: Blueberry Cupcakes

In the second phase, feel free to choose your favourite combination of meals! This is just a sample to give you an idea!

Conclusion

Here we are at the end of this wonderful journey! But hey, your journey is starting right now!...How do you feel? Do you feel excited? Yes, me too!

Remember, keep on going and never quit, the best things come to those who are patient and persevere despite the difficulties. You'll find out that this diet is much easier than you think! Do not only focus on results but enjoy the journey! This is the best way to get the most out of this program!

I really care about your goals and your desire of losing weight and burning fat; that's why I wrote this book. That's why I did my very best and I really hope you appreciate it!

I wish you all the best.

Patricia Garner

CPSIA information can be obtained
at www.ICGtesting.com
Printed in the USA
LVHW060135281020
669972LV00030B/1252